THE TOP 100
FOODS FOR
A YOUNGER YOU

THE TOP 100
FOODS FOR
A YOUNGER YOU

SARAH MERSON

INDEX
BOOKS LTD

The Top 100 Foods for a Younger You
Sarah Merson

First published in the United Kingdom and Ireland in 2007 by
Duncan Baird Publishers Ltd
Sixth Floor, Castle House
75–76 Wells Street, London W1T 3QH

Conceived, created and designed by
Duncan Baird Publishers

This edition published 2007 for Index Books Ltd

Managing Editor: Grace Cheetham
Editor: Ingrid Court-Jones
Managing Designer: Suzanne Tuhrim
Designer: Gail Jones
Commissioned photography: Simon Smith and Toby Scott

British Library Cataloguing-in-Publication Data:
A CIP record for this book is available from the British Library

ISBN: 978-1-84483-556-0

10 9 8 7 6 5 4 3 2 1

Typeset in Helvetica Condensed
Colour reproduction by Colourscan, Singapore
Printed in Thailand by Imago

Publisher's Note: The information in this book is not intended as a substitute for professional medical treatment and advice. The publishers and author cannot accept responsibility for any damage incurred as a result of any of the therapeutic methods contained in this work. The therapeutic methods contained in this book are intended for adult use only. It is advisable to consult a medical professional before using any of these methods, particularly if you are pregnant, breastfeeding or suffering from a medical condition and are unsure of the suitability of any of the remedies or foods mentioned in this book. All recipes serve four unless otherwise specified.

CONTENTS

KEY TO FOOD BENEFITS

Brain power

Hair, teeth and nails

Skin

Eyes

Heart and circulation

Musculo-skeletal system

Immune system

Energy levels

Introduction

We're living longer today than ever before. Not only this, but our expectations for health and well-being are also greater. We are no longer willing to accept the inevitability of the ageing process – instead, we're striving for a fitter, healthier and more youthful existence. And, it's not only about *feeling* great, but about *looking* great, too.

For centuries we've accepted that our appearance will deteriorate as the years go by, but science is now proving that the food we eat can put the brakes on the ageing process, both on the inside and on the outside. It's long been established that a healthy diet is the cornerstone of a long life, and now we're realizing that it's the key to a youthful life as well. Luckily, eating good food is one of life's great pleasures, and if we invest in a healthy diet now, we can help to prevent ourselves from suffering in later years from ailments such as deteriorating eyesight, arthritis and heart disease, as well as fatigue, wrinkles and lacklustre skin.

To get the most from our diet, it's vital to

choose food with integrity – fresh, natural and unadulterated produce is best. By combining fruits, vegetables, nuts, seeds, whole grains, meat, fish, eggs, dairy products, herbs and spices with plenty of water, we achieve a diet full of life-enhancing nutrients. These give the body the necessary means to keep healthy and to function efficiently, which in turn help us to feel fitter and look younger.

Certain foods, especially fruits and vegetables, are powerful sources of free radical-fighting antioxidants. Many of the visible effects of ageing, such as wrinkles, and also those that we can't see, such as deterioration of the heart and eyes, are caused by free radicals – highly reactive molecules

EAT YOURSELF YOUNGER

EAT OR DRINK MORE ...
- **Foods loaded with vitamin C** to counteract free-radical damage and maintain a glowing complexion
- **Selenium-rich foods** to avoid wrinkles, offer protection against damage from the sun, and promote glossy hair
- **Foods containing iron** to prevent lacklustre hair and a pale complexion
- **Vitamin B-rich foods** to increase brain power and maintain the nervous system
- **Foods high in calcium** to help to preserve bone health

- **Foods rich in B, C and E vitamins** to maintain a strong immune system
- **Foods containing zinc** to slow hair loss and promote hair growth
- **Calcium-, magnesium-, boron- or silica-rich foods** to treat fragile, splitting nails
- **Foods high in vitamin A** to boost immunity and maintain glowing skin and sparkling, healthy eyes
- **Foods containing silica** for healthy skin, bones and connective tissue
- **Foods high in vitamin E** for its ability to heal and moisturize the

skin, prevent memory loss and protect the heart
- **Potassium-rich foods** to reduce high blood pressure and maintain a regular heartbeat
- **Foods high in sulphur (a constituent of keratin and collagen)** to promote healthy skin, nails and hair
- **Foods with a low glycaemic index (G.I.)** for a sustained release of energy
- **Foods containing omega-3 and omega-6 essential fatty acids** for an alert brain, clear, glowing skin and protection against heart disease

**STAR FOODS FOR
A YOUNGER YOU:**
grape *see pages 10–11*
avocado *see pages 34–5*
almond *see pages 60–61*
barley *see pages 70–71*
soya bean *see pages 78–9*
sardine *see pages 82–3*
egg *see pages 92–3*
green tea *see pages 96–7*
water *see pages 110–111*
olive oil *see pages 118–119*

that damage cell walls and the genetic material within cells. Free radicals are hard to avoid as they're produced naturally in the course of everyday life – factors such as smoking, pollution and overexposure to sunlight can accelerate their production. However, eating lots of antioxidant-rich fruits and vegetables can be a powerful defence against them and the damage they cause. For example, studies show that eating citrus fruit, which is full of the well-known antioxidant vitamin C, can help to boost the immune system, promote healthy skin and reduce the risk of eye disease. And eating green leafy vegetables, orange sweet potatoes, and apricots and pumpkin, which are all rich in beta-carotene, can help to maintain good eyesight, as well as protect against heart disease.

Foods that are rich in essential fatty acids (EFAs), especially fish, nuts and seeds also play a vital role in helping us to feel and to look fantastic. Not only do EFAs play a central role in keeping the brain active, the mind agile and the nervous system healthy, but they are also fundamental to the preservation of the elasticity of the skin and to keeping the hair glossy and healthy.

Many other foods and herbs can be used to maintain the skin and the hair in tip-top condition, not only by eating them, but also by using them topically. For example, a milk bath is highly nourishing and helps to keep the skin soft and supple; green tea applied to the area around the eyes helps to reduce sagging, while banana acts as a fantastic hair conditioner.

True, ageing is inevitable, but ageing gracefully is an art that anyone can master. Armed with the information in this book, you can use everyday foods and herbs to boost your energy levels and improve both your physical and mental performances. This is all achievable in the short term and you will soon see and feel results. In the longer term, you will benefit by staying fitter, feeling better and looking younger. So don't delay – *now* is the time to invest in your future health and good looks.

FOR A YOUNGER YOU AVOID ...

- junk foods
- sugar
- too much salt
- too much alcohol
- smoking
- stress
- lack of exercise
- lack of sleep

grape

NUTRIENTS
B-vitamins, vitamin C; iron,
potassium, selenium, zinc;
anthocyanins, flavones, quercetin;
fibre

A great source of instant energy, succulent grapes
provide all-round protection.

Grapes contain an enormous number of compounds that are
uniquely nourishing, thus giving them a reputation as a food
for convalescents. This aromatic fruit can prevent and help to
treat any number of age-related conditions, from anaemia and
fatigue to arthritis, varicose veins and rheumatism.

GRAPE JUICE

**2.7kg/6lb ripe black grapes
piece of muslin**

Wash the grapes and collect
them in a large stockpot.
Mash them so that the juice
begins to flow. Cover them
with water and bring to the
boil, then reduce to simmer for
10 minutes. Mash them again,
breaking up as many grapes
as possible. Then, secure the
muslin over another pot and
pour the juice through it.
Allow juice to stand overnight.
Remove muslin and drink.

HELP FOR THE HEART

Full of powerful antioxidants, including astringent tannins,
flavones and anthocyanins, grapes help to prevent "bad" LDL
cholesterol from oxidizing and blood from clotting, and
therefore protect the heart and the circulatory system. High in
both water and fibre, grapes are a great aid for detoxifying the
gut and the liver. Black grapes also contain quercetin, which
helps to minimize inflammation, aiding the cardiovascular
system further, as well as promoting healthy digestion.

Since the earliest times, grapes have been dried to make
raisins. Dynamos of concentrated nutrients, raisins are full of
fibre and are an exceptionally high-energy food. They are also
rich in the minerals iron, potassium, selenium and zinc.
Selenium, in particular, is a very important anti-ageing nutrient,

offering protection from heart disease and boosting the immune system. In addition, selenium helps the skin by keeping fine lines and wrinkles at bay.

GRAPE FACE CREAM

handful of grapes
1 tbsp fresh double cream
½ tsp lemon juice

Crush the grapes with a fork and press through a sieve to extract 1 tablespoonful of juice. Beat the cream and grape juice together to form a light, fluffy cream. Add the lemon juice gradually, stirring gently and mixing well. Apply to the face and neck. Leave for 10 minutes, then rinse off with warm water.

mango

NUTRIENTS
Vitamins C, E, beta-carotene; fibre

.High in vitamin C and beta-carotene, mangoes protect against premature ageing in many ways.

An average-sized mango contains almost the total recommended daily allowance of the antioxidant vitamin C, which produces collagen – a protein central to healthy skin and connective tissue. Mango is also one of the few fruit sources of vitamin E, which together with vitamin C, protects the brain from memory loss. With bright orange-yellow flesh, mangoes are high in beta-carotene, which is needed for clear skin, healthy lungs, a strong heart and good overall immunity.

MANGO LASSI

500g/1lb 2oz natural yoghurt
1½ mangoes, peeled and
   sliced
55g/2oz/¼ cup caster sugar
8 ice cubes
4 pistachios, shelled
4 almonds
pinch of saffron threads

Blend the yoghurt, mango, sugar and ice until frothy. Cut the pistachios and almonds into slivers. Pour the lassi into glasses and garnish with the nuts and saffron threads.

apricot

With their high carotenoid content, apricots contain a wealth of youth-enhancing nutrients.

Beta-carotene is the most abundant antioxidant found in apricots, helping to protect the skin and lungs from oxidation damage and supporting the immune system. It also prevents free radicals from damaging the eyes. In addition, apricots contain lycopene, one of the most powerful antioxidants. Lycopene is known for its ability to prevent the build-up of fatty deposits in the arteries and it also has strong anti-carcinogenic properties.

NUTRIENTS
B-vitamins, vitamin C, beta-carotene, lycopene; iron; fibre

BRANDIED APRICOTS

2kg/4lb 8oz fresh apricots
bag of cloves
4 cinnamon sticks
1.3kg/3lb brown sugar
600ml/21fl oz/2½ cups vinegar
60ml/2fl oz/4 tbsp brandy

Wash the apricots and stick 2–3 cloves into each one. In a saucepan combine the cinnamon sticks, sugar and vinegar; bring to the boil, and simmer to form a syrup. Put the apricots in the syrup and continue to simmer until soft. Remove from the heat and pack apricots into jars. Add 1 tablespoonful of brandy and a cinnamon stick to each jar, and seal. The apricots will be ready to eat after 14 days.

blueberry

Blueberries contain great youth-preserving antioxidants, which stave off many conditions.

Blueberries are a rich source of anthocyanin, a potent antioxidant that protects against ageing and improves circulation. Anthocyanin also increases the potency of vitamin C, thus supporting collagen and improving the skin. Blueberries help to improve brain function, as well as to fight eye disease. They are also a good source of pectin, which lowers cholesterol levels. Topically, their fruit acid content helps them to act as a gentle astringent and peeling agent.

NUTRIENTS
Vitamins C, E, beta-carotene; anthocyanin, ellagic acid; fibre

Blueberries are popularly known as "brain berries" because they protect the brain from ageing.

BLUEBERRY SAUCE

250g/9oz/2 cups fresh
  blueberries
80g/2¾oz/⅓ cup sugar
1 tbsp fresh lemon juice
pinch of salt
½ tsp vanilla extract

Wash the blueberries and crush them in a bowl. Add the sugar, lemon juice and salt. Mix well. In a saucepan heat the mixture and boil for 1 minute. Add the vanilla extract. Serve with puddings, cake or ice cream. Keeps in the fridge for 5 days.

papaya

Full of beta-carotene and vitamin C, papaya also contains papain, a powerful anti-ageing enzyme.

With plenty of beta-carotene and vitamin C, papaya helps to reduce deterioration of the arteries and lessen the risk of heart disease, as well as fight free radicals. Papaya is also rich in papain, which acts as a wonderful digestive aid that encourages the elimination of waste products. It's also useful for calming inflammation throughout the body. Used topically, papain literally digests dead skin cells and acts as an excellent mild exfoliant.

NUTRIENTS
Vitamin C, beta-carotene, folic acid; potassium; papain; fibre

PAPAYA EXFOLIATING LOTION *(to brighten and rejuvenate the skin)*

1 large fresh papaya
piece of muslin
1 cup chamomile infusion,
  cooled

Peel the papaya, remove the seeds and purée the flesh in a food processor or blender. Press the purée through a piece of muslin to extract all the juice. Mix the juice with an equal amount of chamomile infusion, and stir well. Using cotton wool balls, apply the lotion to the face and neck, avoiding contact with the eyes. Leave for about 10 minutes, then rinse off. Keeps in the fridge for up to 2 days.

orange

NUTRIENTS
B-vitamins, vitamin C, carotenoids, folic acid; potassium; limonene; fibre

VITAMIN C SMOOTHIE

700ml/24fl oz/3 cups freshly squeezed orange juice
450g/1lb fresh mango chunks
450g/1lb fresh strawberries
450g/1lb kiwi fruit, chopped
500ml/17fl oz vanilla yoghurt
crushed ice (optional)

Combine all the ingredients in a blender and whizz until smooth. Add ice as required, then pour into tumblers.

As well as vitamin C, oranges contain hesperidin, a key antioxidant for a healthy heart.

Rich in Vitamin C, oranges help to maintain healthy, youthful skin, prevent eye problems, and stop free radicals from clogging up the arteries, a key risk factor for heart disease. Containing the antioxidant hesperidin, oranges are said to protect the heart further by raising healthy HDL cholesterol and lowering "bad" LDL cholesterol. The fruits also contain limonene, which has anti-carcinogenic properties. They provide natural sugars to boost flagging energy levels, are high in fibre and are even reputed to reduce cellulite.

cranberry

Cranberries are high in a number of compounds that stave off age-related conditions.

Cranberries contain ellagic acid, which is an antioxidant compound that has been shown to disarm carcinogens, as well as prevent the onset of heart disease. This antioxidant is best absorbed from food in its natural state – good news for those who enjoy eating cranberries. Packed with vitamin C, cranberries are also excellent for keeping the skin and eyes youthful, and for boosting immunity. The berries contain two other ingredients that help to stave off heart disease – the powerful bioflavonoids quercetin and myrcetin.

NUTRIENTS
Vitamin C; iron; ellagic acid; tannins

CHOCOLATE-COVERED CRANBERRIES

350g/12oz milk chocolate chips
2 tbsp butter
350g/12oz fresh cranberries

Melt the chocolate chips and butter over a low heat, stirring frequently until melted. Using a toothpick, dip the cranberries in the chocolate until they are coated. Lay them out on wax paper. Refrigerate until hard.

lemon

NUTRIENTS
Vitamin C, folic acid; potassium; limonene; fibre

Whether ingested or used topically, lemons provide a wealth of youth-preserving properties.

The high level of vitamin C in lemons means that they are vital for healthy skin and gums. They are also a good source of bioflavonoids, such as quercetin, which boost the effects of vitamin C, and are particularly important for the health of blood vessels and to prevent varicose veins. Lemons, as with other citrus fruits, contain terpenes, which are anti-carcinogenic. When used in beauty treatments, lemon juice inhibits bacterial growth and is astringent, strengthening and toning.

LEMON TONER
(to treat thread veins)

**4 tsp vegetable glycerin
juice of 1 lemon
1 drop neroli essential oil
1 drop rose essential oil**

Mix the vegetable glycerin with the lemon juice and add the essential oils. Apply twice daily to thread veins. Keeps in a sealed jar for up to 3 months.

600

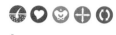

banana

One of the most nourishing fruits, bananas contain many important anti-ageing nutrients.

Bananas are high in potassium, which keeps high blood pressure in check and reduces the risk of heart disease. Potassium works with sodium to maintain the fluid and electrolyte balance in body cells, so bananas help to maintain healthy nerve and muscle function. They have FOS (fructo-oligo-saccharides) to help to feed "good" bacteria in the gut, and aid digestion. They also contain tryptophan, which the body converts to serotonin to aid peaceful sleep.

NUTRIENTS
Vitamins B3, B5, B6; magnesium, potassium; fibre

To ripen bananas, put them in a brown paper bag and keep at room temperature.

BANANA CONDITIONER
(to moisturize dry hair)

1 ripe banana
2 tsp grapeseed oil

Mash the banana using a fork, then mix with the oil to make a paste. Massage into the hair and scalp, then cover the hair with cling film and leave for 30 minutes. Wash out, using a mild shampoo.

prune

Prunes are full of antioxidant power and are great for slowing down the ageing process.

Prunes have long been known as a rich source of fibre, but weight for weight, they are the most potent of all antioxidant foods. Their high level of potassium keeps blood pressure in check, while their vitamin B6 protects the heart and boosts brain power. Prunes are also full of iron, providing energy and preventing fatigue. The combination of iron and vitamin A is especially good for hair growth, while vitamin A itself maintains youthful skin and eyes.

NUTRIENTS
Vitamins A, B3, B6; potassium, iron; fibre

PRUNE WHIP

12 large prunes
3 egg whites
3 tbsp caster sugar

Preheat the oven to 300°F/ 150°C/Gas mark 2. Soak the prunes overnight and stew in the soaking water until tender. Remove stones and mash to a smooth pulp. Beat the egg whites until stiff, fold in the sugar and then the prune pulp. Turn into a greased dish and bake for about 20 minutes. Serve with cream.

kiwi fruit

Kiwi fruit contain almost twice as much vitamin C as oranges, and more fibre than apples.

With their high levels of vitamin C, kiwi fruit are a great immunity booster and are particularly good for preserving youthful skin. They are loaded with lutein, a carotene, which, together with vitamins C and E, helps to reduce blood clotting as well as blood fats. Kiwi fruit are also potassium-rich, preventing many age-related conditions from high blood pressure to insomnia and exhaustion. Their fibre content promotes effective digestion and helps to lower cholesterol.

NUTRIENTS
Vitamins B3, C, E, lutein; potassium; fibre

KIWI FRUIT ICE

4 kiwi fruit, peeled and chopped
500ml/17fl oz/2 cups unsweetened apple juice
1 tbsp lemon juice
½ tsp grated orange rind

Combine the kiwi fruit, apple juice and lemon juice in a blender, and whizz until smooth. Stir in the orange rind. Pour mixture into a 20cm/8in tray and freeze until almost firm. Spoon the frozen mixture into a mixing bowl, and beat until fluffy. Return the mixture to the tray, and freeze again until firm. Leave out at room temperature for about 10 minutes before serving.

blackcurrant

NUTRIENTS
Vitamin C; potassium, magnesium; bioflavonoids; fibre

Blackcurrants contain a host of powerful anti-ageing nutrients, particularly vitamin C.

Blackcurrants are an extraordinary source of vitamin C, containing four times as much as the equivalent weight of oranges. Well-known for attacking free radicals, vitamin C boosts the body's defences, and promotes tissue and cell repair, as well as growth. These tiny berries also contain bioflavonoids, which improve the condition of blood vessels and the skin. In addition, the large amount of potassium in blackcurrants treats water retention and high blood pressure.

BLACKCURRANT TONER *(to combat wrinkles)*

60g/2¼oz/½ cup blackcurrants
piece of muslin
10 grapes
1 tbsp fresh lemon juice

Whizz the blackcurrants in a blender and strain them through muslin. Reserve 75ml/2¾fl oz of the juice. Repeat the procedure with the grapes and save the same amount of juice. Mix together the blackcurrant and grape juices, add the lemon juice and pour into a bottle. Apply to the face and neck twice daily with cotton wool balls, leaving to dry naturally. Seal the bottle and store in the fridge for 48 hours.

blackberry

Plump, sweet and juicy, blackberries are one of the richest low-fat sources of vitamin E.

Like most berries, blackberries are an excellent source of vitamin C, but what sets them apart is that they also contain good amounts of vitamin E. This helps to neutralize free radicals, which cause heart disease and premature ageing of the skin. Blackberries are also a natural source of salicylate, the active substance found in aspirin, which helps the body to fight infection. Some studies have shown that salicylate also has anti-carcinogenic properties.

NUTRIENTS
Vitamins C, E, folic acid; manganese; salicylate; flavonoids

Add blackberries to your breakfast cereal to help your body to absorb iron from the cereal.

BLACKBERRY AND APPLE FOOL

4 Bramley cooking apples
2 tbsp caster sugar
300g/10oz/2½ cups blackberries
625ml/22fl oz/2½ cups
bio-yoghurt

Peel and slice the apples and put in a saucepan with the sugar. Heat gently until soft. Stir in the blackberries and cook for a further 1–2 minutes. Allow the mixture to cool, then stir in the yoghurt. Chill in the fridge.

Cantaloupe melon

NUTRIENTS
Vitamins B3, C, beta-carotene; potassium

These succulent summer fruits are bursting with antioxidants to fight ageing free radicals.

Cantaloupe melons are very high in vitamin C and beta-carotene, both of which are naturally anti-ageing and aid cell repair and growth, as well as supporting the immune and circulatory systems. Cantaloupes also contain potassium, which can lower high blood pressure and "bad" LDL cholesterol. With their high water content, cantaloupes help to detoxify the body.

MELON LOTION
(to cool and hydrate the skin)

¼ **fresh melon, peeled and deseeded**
piece of muslin
½ **lemon**
1 tbsp olive oil

Whizz the melon in a blender, then filter the juice through the muslin. Squeeze the lemon to extract 1 teaspoonful of juice. Combine the melon juice, lemon juice and olive oil in a container, cover and store in the fridge. Apply twice daily to the face and neck with cotton wool. Keeps in the fridge for up to 2 days.

apple

Containing fibre, flavonoids and vitamin C, apples are a healthy addition to any anti-ageing diet.

Apples contain pectin, a fibre that flushes waste products out of the body. It also encourages beneficial bacteria to proliferate in the gut and, with quercetin, helps to keep cholesterol levels down. Apples contain malic acid, too, which relieves rheumatism and arthritis, and assists with energy production. The fruits' vitamin C boosts immunity, while their high water content rehydrates the body.

NUTRIENTS
Vitamin C; malic acid, flavonoids; fibre

Avoid commercial apple juice drinks because they contain high amounts of sugar.

APPLE, PEAR AND MINT JUICE *(to aid digestion)*

8 apples, cored
8 pears, cored
12 stems of fresh mint

Wash all the fruit, then cut it into chunks, leaving the skin on. Feed through a juicer with the mint. Pour into large glasses and drink immediately.

pineapple

NUTRIENTS
Vitamins B1, B2, C; manganese; bromelain; fibre

Pineapple is particularly rich in bromelain, which helps to reduce inflammation in the body.

Pineapple's main benefits come from bromelain, which is an effective anti-inflammatory, making it exceptionally good for joint problems. Rich in vitamin C, pineapple supports the immune system and defends against free radicals, which can cause premature ageing. It's also an excellent source of manganese – an essential co-factor in a number of enzymes important for antioxidant defences and energy production.

PINEAPPLE AND MANGO SALSA

1 large ripe mango
½ small pineapple
¼ red onion
1cm piece fresh root ginger, peeled and grated
1 small clove garlic, peeled and crushed
½ small red chilli, finely sliced
handful of coriander, roughly chopped
juice of 2 limes
1 tsp sesame oil

Peel and chop the flesh of the fruits, then put it in a bowl with the onion, ginger, garlic, chilli and coriander. Toss well. Drizzle the lime juice and sesame oil on to the mixture. Serve with fish or chicken, or as a dip.

017

grapefruit

The perfect breakfast food, grapefruit is loaded with antioxidants and is a powerful detoxifier.

Grapefruit is a rich source of youth-preserving vitamin C. The pink variety, in particular, is a good source of potassium and bioflavonoids, both of which are important for the heart and circulation, as well as the skin and immunity. The pectin content helps to eliminate cholesterol from the body. Grapefruit is also rich in alpha-hydroxy-acids (AHAs), which make it an effective toner when used topically.

NUTRIENTS
Vitamin C, beta-carotene, folic acid, lycopene; potassium; flavonoids; fibre

GRAPEFRUIT BEAUTY MASK *(to tone the skin)*

1 small grapefruit
1 small pot natural yoghurt

Peel the grapefruit and break it into segments. Remove the pith and pips, and combine with the yoghurt in a blender. Whizz to make a paste. Put the mixture in a bowl and leave in the fridge for 1 hour. Apply to the face and leave for about 10 minutes. Gently remove with cool water.

018

strawberry

One of the delights of summer, strawberries are full of age-defying nutrients.

NUTRIENTS
Vitamins B6, C, folic acid; ellagic acid

Strawberries are an excellent source of vitamin C, which is essential for the manufacture of collagen – a protein that helps to maintain the structure of the skin. Vitamin C also plays an important role in healing wounds and can ward off gingivitis, the gum disease that affects three out of four adults. Strawberries also contain ellagic acid, a phytochemical that has powerful anti-carcinogenic properties.

Stop strawberries from going soggy by hulling them immediately after washing them.

STRAWBERRY AND RICOTTA SPREAD

150g/6oz/1 cup ripe
  strawberries
2 limes
2 tsp icing sugar
100g/3oz/⅓ cup ricotta cheese

Mash the strawberries with a fork and grate the zest of the limes. Add the icing sugar and the lime zest and stir well into the ricotta cheese to form a smooth mixture. Spread over toasted cinnamon bagels for a delicious breakfast treat.

raspberry

Raspberries are loaded with vitamin C and many potent antioxidants that keep us young.

The high vitamin C content in raspberries boosts immunity and can help to prevent everything from heart disease to eye problems. The fruits also contain ellagic acid, which is anti-carcinogenic and prevents adverse cellular changes. The anthocyanins in raspberries have anti-inflammatory properties, thus protecting from conditions such as arthritis. Raspberries are also effective in combating a number of viruses and bacteria. In addition, they are one of the top fruit sources of fibre, therefore improving digestion.

NUTRIENTS
Vitamins B3, C, folic acid; iron, manganese; flavonoids, anthocyanins; fibre

RASPBERRY SYLLABUB

225g/8oz/1¼ cups raspberries
150ml/5fl oz/⅔ cup dry sherry, or dry white wine
2 tbsp brandy
grated rind of 1 orange
grated rind of ½ lemon
75g/3oz/⅓ cup sugar
450ml/15½fl oz/2 cups double cream

Crush the raspberries slightly (leaving 2 handfuls aside for serving) and mix in a bowl with the other ingredients except the cream. Marinate for 4 hours, then force the mixture through a sieve. Add the cream and whip to soft peaks. Put the reserved raspberries in serving glasses; top with mixture and chill. Serve with brandy snaps.

fig

NUTRIENTS
Vitamin B6, beta-carotene;
potassium, iron; fibre

Figs are a fabulous source of fibre. They also add hard-to-come-by vitamin B6 to the diet.

High in fibre, figs can encourage the elimination of toxins and help to lower the risk of heart disease. They are a good source of potassium, which is crucial for controlling blood pressure and lowering the risk of developing heart conditions. Figs also provide useful amounts of vitamin B6, without which we can suffer from a poor memory and increased stress levels.

FIGS STUFFED WITH ORANGE-ANISE CREAM

16 dried figs
115g/4 oz/½ cup cream cheese, at room temperature
1 tbsp fresh orange juice
2 tsp grated orange rind
1½ tsp honey
½ tsp aniseed, crushed

Trim and discard the stems from the figs. Cut an "X" down through the stem ends and gently push each fig open. In a bowl combine the cream cheese, orange juice, orange rind, honey and aniseed. Beat until creamy. Spoon a dollop of mixture into each fig. Keeps in the fridge for up to 2 hours.

pomegranate

Pomegranates are one of the most powerful sources of antioxidants among fruits.

Extremely high in ellagic acid, pomegranates have anti-carcinogenic and anti-heart disease properties. Antioxidants in pomegranates protect against free-radical damage, including to the skin, and also keep the arteries clear. The antioxidant chemicals also help to protect the skin from sun damage.

NUTRIENTS
Vitamins B1, B3, C; calcium, phosphorus; ellagic acid

POMEGRANATE PUNCH

5 or 6 pomegranates
250g/9oz/1 cup sugar
500ml/18fl oz water
250ml/9fl oz/1 cup fresh
    orange juice
60ml/2 fl oz/¼ cup fresh
    lemon juice
1 litre/35fl oz/4 cups ginger
    ale

Scoop out the pomegranate seeds and put them through a juicer. In a large jug dissolve the sugar in the water by stirring rapidly. Add the juiced pomegranate, orange and lemon juices, then the ginger ale. Chill in the fridge and serve.

cherry

Cherries are packed with antioxidants that have amazing anti-ageing properties.

Cherries are rich in flavonoids such as anthocyanins, which the body uses to help boost immunity. They also contain quercetin, a strong anti-inflammatory substance, which helps to relieve painful joints and protects against eye disease. Cherries are also rich in the phytochemical ellagic acid, which has anti-carcinogenic properties, and vitamin C, which strengthens collagen and maintains healthy-looking skin and hair. In addition, vitamin C aids the fight against viruses and bacteria.

CHERRY ICE CREAM SUNDAE

6 tbsp caramel ice-cream topping
60ml/2fl oz/¼ cup Grand Marnier
500ml/17fl oz/2 cups vanilla ice cream
225g/8oz cherries, pitted
handful of crushed biscuit crumbs

Combine the ice-cream topping and Grand Marnier in a small dish, stirring until smooth. Divide the ice cream among 4 dessert bowls. Top with the cherries, add the sauce and biscuit crumbs, and serve.

rhubarb

A vegetable "fruit", rhubarb is a fantastic source of dietary fibre as well as vitamin C and minerals.

NUTRIENTS
Vitamin C; calcium, magnesium, potassium; oxalic acid; fibre

Full of fibre, rhubarb acts as a natural food laxative, keeping the digestive system in good working order and helping to lower cholesterol and prevent heart disease. It's a good source of immunity-supporting vitamin C, which also helps to plump out wrinkles and keep the skin from premature ageing. Rhubarb is high in calcium for the bones, and potassium to keep blood pressure in check and protect the heart. It is also extremely high in water, which helps to keep the body well hydrated.

RHUBARB FROZEN YOGHURT

300g/10½ oz/2 cups stewed rhubarb
100g/3½oz/½ cup natural low-fat yoghurt
3 tbsp granulated sugar
2 tbsp orange juice

In a food processor purée the stewed rhubarb until smooth.

Blend in the yoghurt, sugar and orange juice. Cover and freeze in a shallow metal pan for 3–4 hours or until almost firm. Break up the mixture and whizz again in the food processor until smooth. Freeze in an airtight container for 1 hour or until the mixture is firm.

avocado

NUTRIENTS
B-vitamins, vitamins C, E,
carotenoids; potassium, zinc;
beta-sitosterol

Full of vitamins A, B, C and E and essential fatty acids, avocado fights free radicals and is highly nourishing for the skin.

Avocado is native to Central America, and is now grown in tropical regions throughout the world.

ANTIOXIDANT POWER

Loaded with vitamins C and E, avocados are excellent for keeping the skin soft, supple and healthy, and for maintaining glossy hair. They are high in omega-3 fatty acids, thus helping to prevent wrinkles, enhance brain power and treat arthritic pain. Avocados are also high in oleic acid, the building block for omega-9 fatty acids, which are also excellent for the skin and have anti-inflammatory properties. They have high levels of the antioxidant lutein, which studies have shown to help protect against eye problems and cardiovascular disease.

HEART HEALTHY

With their smooth buttery texture, avocados are high in monounsaturated fat, which raises levels of "good" cholesterol while slightly lowering fatty triglycerides, and beta-sitosterol, a phytonutrient that lowers "bad" cholesterol. They're also full of

---

AVOCADO AND BABY SPINACH SALAD

2 ripe avocados, stoned, peeled and cubed
16 cherry tomatoes, halved
2 handfuls of baby spinach, washed and torn into pieces

For the dressing:
juice of 2 limes
2 tsp honey
pinch of salt

Make the dressing by combining the ingredients in a jug, and shaking well. Put all the salad ingredients in a bowl and coat with the dressing. Mix gently and serve immediately.

fibre, and are a source of linoleic acid, which the body converts to gamma-linolenic acid (GLA), a substance that helps to thin the blood. Avocados are also one of the richest sources of potassium, which is essential for healthy blood pressure and muscle contraction.

AVOCADO FACE PACK
(to rejuvenate tired skin)

1 ripe avocado
1 tsp clear honey
1 tsp lemon juice
1 tsp natural yoghurt

Combine all the ingredients in a bowl and mash into a paste. Leave in the fridge for 30 minutes. Apply the pack to your face and leave for 10 minutes before removing with cool water.

beetroot

Vibrant in colour, beetroot is loaded with nutrients to help us look younger and feel better.

Containing the powerful antioxidant betacyanin, which gives beetroot its deep red hue, this vegetable purifies the blood and has anti-carcinogenic properties. Research shows that beetroot boosts the body's natural defences in the liver, regenerating immune cells. It also helps to lower cholesterol levels'. In addition, beetroot contains silica, which is vital for healthy skin, hair, fingernails, ligaments, tendons and bones.

NUTRIENTS
Iron, manganese, potassium, silica; betacyanin; fibre,

GINGERED BEETROOT

4 beetroot (with tops), scrubbed and chopped
2 tsp sesame seeds
1 tbsp light soy sauce
1 tbsp extra virgin olive oil
1 tbsp ginger root, finely chopped
100g/3½oz/¾ cup grated carrots

Steam the beetroot over a high heat for 30–40 minutes until tender. Steam the tops for 3–4 minutes, until wilted. Meanwhile, toast the sesame seeds in a dry pan until browned. Then, in a bowl, whisk together the soy sauce, olive oil and ginger, add all the other ingredients and toss well. Serve warm, or as a salad dish.

cucumber

Laden with water, this popular salad vegetable is well known for its skin-healing properties.

Used topically, cucumber helps to maintain a youthful appearance, thanks to its hydrating and anti-inflammatory properties. When ingested, the high water and balanced mineral content makes it one of the best diuretics. Cucumbers are a rich source of silica, a mineral needed for healthy skin, bone and connective tissue. Silica also plays a major role in preventing cardiovascular disease and osteoporosis.

NUTRIENTS
Vitamins A, C; magnesium, manganese, potassium, silica; fibre

CUCUMBER CLEANSER
(to refresh and revive the skin)

½ small cucumber
5 mint leaves
60ml/2fl oz/¼ cup milk
2 drops grapefruit seed extract

Peel and chop the cucumber. Remove the mint leaves from their stalks and chop. Put both in a food processor with the milk and whizz until smooth. Pour the mixture into a saucepan and bring to the boil. Reduce heat and simmer for 2 minutes, then allow to cool. Pour into a clean bottle and add the grapefruit seed extract. Store in the fridge and use within a week.

celery

Containing very few calories, celery aids weight loss and keeps us looking young.

NUTRIENTS
Folic acid, beta-carotene; potassium

It is believed that we burn more calories chewing, swallowing and digesting celery, than we get from eating it, making the vegetable popular with dieters. Its high water content acts as a diuretic helping to eliminate puffy hands, ankles and feet. Celery is also excellent for the body's detoxifying processes, including cleansing of the liver, which helps to keep skin looking youthful.

100g of celery contains only 7 calories, so it's an ideal food for weight watchers

CELERY RAGOÛT

20g/¾ oz butter
1 head celery, sliced
400g/14oz carrots, peeled and
    sliced
1 red onion, sliced

Melt the butter in a saucepan. Add the vegetables and coat them in the butter. Season to taste. Cover and cook over a very low heat for 30–40 minutes, shaking often to avoid sticking. Serve with grilled fish.

pepper

When fully ripe, peppers are a terrific source
of vitamin C and other anti-ageing antioxidants.

NUTRIENTS
Vitamin C, beta-carotene, lycopene;
fibre

Peppers are packed with vitamin C, which helps to fight almost
every aspect of the ageing process, including deterioration of
the skin structure and damage to the arteries. Vitamin C is said
to quash carcinogenic free radicals, and to protect against
memory problems and eye disease. It is also a potent
immunity booster. Red peppers are a rich source of lycopene,
another renowned anti-carcinogenic nutrient.

ROAST PEPPER AND BASIL DIP

1 large red pepper
100ml/4fl oz/nearly ½ cup milk
½ tsp paprika
½ tsp salt
2 tsps extra virgin olive oil
2 tsps cider vinegar
1 tbsp basil, chopped

Preheat the oven to 200°C/
400°F/Gas mark 6. Put the
whole pepper on a baking tray in

the centre of the oven for 20–30
minutes, or until the skin goes
black. Remove, and allow to
cool. Peel off the skin, seed
and core, and save any juice.
Blend all the ingredients,
including the pepper and its
juice, in a food processor to
a smooth creamy texture. Serve
either chilled as a dip, or warm
as a sauce.

parsnip

NUTRIENTS

B-vitamins, vitamin E, folic acid; potassium, silica; fibre

Parsnip contains a host of nutrients recognized for their youth-promoting and beautifying effects.

Parsnips are a valuable source of potassium, B-vitamins, vitamin E and trace minerals such as silica, as well as fibre. Potassium reduces high blood pressure, while folic acid is anti-carcinogenic. Vitamin E has been dubbed "the fountain of youth" for its heart-protective properties and ability to prevent skin damage from sun exposure. Parsnips' silica content strengthens the skin and all connective tissue.

PARSNIP CURRY

½ white onion, chopped
1 tbsp extra virgin olive oil
½ tsp cumin seeds, crushed
1 tsp chilli powder
125ml/4fl oz/½ cup water
450g/1lb parsnips, peeled and cubed
60g/2¼oz green peppers, cut into thin strips
80g/2¾oz/¼ cup peanuts, chopped

Sauté the onion with the spices in the oil for 5–8 minutes. Add the water and parsnips, bring to a boil, cover, and simmer over a low heat for 20–30 minutes until the parsnips are tender but not mushy. Garnish with the peppers and the peanuts before serving.

Parsnips retain more nutrients if kept in the fridge rather than at room temperature.

onion

A cousin of garlic, onion contains powerful antioxidants and is reputed to counter cellulite.

Onions regulate blood pressure and prevent blood cells clumping. They are a rich source of quercetin, which has anti-carcinogenic properties, and they act as an anti-inflammatory. Onions are an excellent source of selenium, which boosts immunity, cleanses the liver and staves off wrinkles and sun damage. They are also a key source of sulphur, a constituent of the building blocks of skin, nails and hair.

NUTRIENTS
B-vitamins; selenium, sulphur; quercetin

FRENCH ONION SOUP

4 tbsp extra virgin olive oil
750g/1½lbs onions, thinly
  sliced
2 cloves garlic, crushed
2 tbsp apple juice
1.2litres/41fl oz/4 cups beef
  stock
300ml/10fl oz dry white wine
salt and pepper, to taste

In a heavy saucepan heat the oil. Add the onions, garlic and apple juice, and cook for 5–6 minutes, stirring constantly. Turn down the heat and cook for about 20 minutes. Pour the stock and wine into the mixture and season with salt and pepper. Bring to a simmer and cook uncovered for 1 hour. Pour into bowls and serve.

endive

Tasty in salads, endive is a great source of water, which keeps skin youthful and hydrated.

Bursting with fibre, endive is extremely useful for helping the digestive system to work efficiently by evacuating toxic wastes, including heavy metals, from the body. Endive is almost 94 per cent water, thus it hydrates the body and improves circulation, benefiting all the organs including the skin and the heart. It's also a diuretic and is very low in calories, so it helps with weight loss.

NUTRIENTS
Vitamin C, beta-carotene; calcium, magnesium; fibre

ENDIVES WITH ROQUEFORT SAUCE

4 endives
100g/3½oz/½ cup Roquefort cheese
200ml/7floz/scant 1 cup single cream
sprig of fresh thyme

Divide the endive leaves lengthways and place them in a serving dish, open-side up. Put the Roquefort in a saucepan, add the cream and stir over low heat until smooth. Pour the sauce over the endive, sprinkle with thyme and serve.

kale

One of the most power-packed vegetables, kale is especially high in anti-ageing antioxidants.

Kale is rich in everything from B-vitamins and carotenoids to a host of anti-ageing and beautifying trace minerals. Its vitamin B6 and B12 content helps to boost brain power and prevent memory loss. Loaded with beta-carotene, it is also one of the best sources of lutein, a carotenoid that helps to prevent eye disease. Kale is a valuable source of calcium for the bones and silica for the skin, hair, teeth and nails. Silica also counteracts the negative effects of aluminium in the body.

NUTRIENTS
B-vitamins, vitamins C, E, beta-carotene, folic acid, lutein; calcium, iron, silica

KALE WITH GARLIC AND RED PEPPER

455ml/16fl oz/2 cups water
450g/1lb kale, chopped
2 tbsp extra virgin olive oil
½ small onion
2 cloves garlic, crushed
½ tsp sea salt
½ tsp freshly ground pepper
¼ tsp crushed red pepper corns

Put the water in a saucepan and bring to the boil. Add the kale and cook for 2 minutes. Drain and press until barely moist. Put the oil in a large pan and sauté the onion and garlic over a low heat for 4–5 minutes. Stir in the kale, salt, black pepper and red pepper corns and cook over a medium heat for 3–4 minutes. Serve at once.

broccoli

NUTRIENTS
B-vitamins, vitamin C, beta-
carotene; calcium, iron, zinc

Broccoli is a rich source of youth-preserving beta-carotene and vitamin C.

With high levels of carotenoids, especially beta-carotene, broccoli has powerful anti-carcinogenic properties, and has been associated with lower rates of both heart and eye disease. As broccoli can increase vitamin A in the body, it also helps to improve various skin conditions. It is a great source of vitamin C, which helps to boost immunity. Broccoli contains calcium, which staves off osteoporosis, and fibre, which keeps the digestive system working smoothly.

CHINESE-STYLE BROCCOLI

600g/1lb 5oz fresh broccoli
100g/3½oz/½ cup tinned,
  sliced water chestnuts
2 tbsp sunflower oil
small piece of ginger, peeled
  and grated
pinch of grated lemon rind
1 tsp soy sauce
125ml/4½fl oz/½ cup water
½ chicken stock cube

Cut the broccoli into florets. Put the water chestnuts, oil, ginger and lemon rind in a saucepan. Heat, add the broccoli and toss for 1 minute. Add the rest of the ingredients. Bring to the boil, then cover and simmer for 5 minutes. Serve immediately.

spinach

Full of iron, calcium and magnesium, spinach is vital for looking young and feeling fit.

Perhaps best known for its iron content, spinach is excellent for oxygenating the blood, generating energy and preventing anaemia. Iron is also especially effective at preventing premature hair loss. Spinach is a rich source of calcium and magnesium, which work together to stave off osteoporosis. Magnesium also relaxes and dilates blood vessels and keeps the muscles flexible. The vitamin C in spinach keeps the skin healthy, while lipoic acid helps to maintain the memory.

NUTRIENTS
B-vitamins, vitamin C, carotenoids; calcium, magnesium, zinc; lipoic acid; fibre

SPINACH AND CRISPY BACON SALAD

450g/1lb/back bacon slices
4 eggs, hard-boiled and shelled
2 handfuls of pecan nuts, chopped
450g/1lb fresh spinach, washed

Cook the bacon under a grill and cut it into bite-size pieces. Slice the eggs and put them in a bowl with the bacon, pecans and spinach. Toss well to combine. Drizzle with salad dressing and serve.

cabbage

NUTRIENTS

Vitamins B3, C, folic acid; calcium, potassium, sulphur

Cabbage contains a range of sulphurous substances and other nutrients to keep us young.

Cabbage is rich in sulphur, which protects the liver and has anti-carcinogenic properties. Sometimes referred to as the "beauty mineral", sulphur is a constituent of keratin, which is vital for strong nails and glossy hair, and collagen, which keeps the skin youthful. The vitamin C in cabbage mops up free radicals. It also contains vitamin B3, folic acid, calcium and potassium.

STIR-FRIED CABBAGE WITH FENNEL SEEDS

1 green cabbage
2 tbsp balsamic vinegar
1 tsp fennel seeds
pinch of cayenne pepper
salt and pepper, to taste

Wash the cabbage and shred it into thin strips. Put the balsamic vinegar in a wok and heat until sizzling. Add the cabbage, fennel seeds, cayenne pepper, and salt and pepper. Cook until the cabbage is softened and slightly browned.

tomato

Full of carotenoids, particularly lycopene, tomatoes have unique anti-carcinogenic powers.

Lycopene neutralizes free radicals before they can cause damage, therefore staving off everything from wrinkles to heart attacks. Studies indicate that lycopene could have twice the anti-carcinogenic punch of beta-carotene. Tomatoes are high in vitamin C, which supports connective tissue in the body and boosts immunity. In addition, tomatoes contain a little iron, which is well absorbed when accompanied by vitamin C, and prevents anaemia and fatigue.

NUTRIENTS
Vitamins B3, C, E, beta-carotene, lycopene; iron, potassium

SPICY GARDEN COCKTAIL

4 vine-ripened tomatoes
4 small cucumbers
8 celery stalks, with leaves
hot chilli sauce, to taste
celery salt, optional
ice cubes

Cut the tomatoes into chunks and the cucumbers into strips. Remove the celery tops from the stalks, reserving 4 to garnish. Feed the tomatoes, cucumbers and celery stalks through a juicer. Coat the rims of 4 tall glasses with celery salt and pour the juice into the glasses. Add the hot sauce to taste and several ice cubes. Stir well. Garnish with celery tops and serve immediately.

watercress

NUTRIENTS
Vitamins B3, B6, C, carotenoids; calcium, iron, magnesium; fibre

Watercress is a highly protective food that helps to strengthen immunity and keep us youthful.

Watercress is rich in vitamin C, thus aiding the regeneration of skin cells, keeping the liver healthy and defences strong. It also contains phenethyl isothiocyanate, a chemical that helps the liver to detoxify and is said to neutralize carcinogenic cells. Watercress is a useful source of iodine – essential for the proper functioning of the thyroid, and vitamin B6 to prevent memory loss. Watercress also helps the release of bile from the gall bladder, which is important for the digestion of fat.

WATERCRESS, ENDIVE AND ORANGE SALAD

4 endives
juice of 1 lemon
200g/7oz watercress, stalks
   removed
4 oranges, peeled
2 carrots, grated
150ml/5fl oz/⅔ cup apple
   juice

Slice the endives, place in a large salad bowl and squeeze over the lemon juice to stop them browning. Roughly chop the watercress and quarter the oranges. Combine them in the bowl with the remaining ingredients, season and toss well. Serve immediately.

038

♥
globe artichoke

Artichokes are a fantastic food for improving digestion and assisting the body to detoxify.

Artichokes contain cynarin, which increases the flow of bile and improves liver function. The result is better digestion and breakdown of all types of fat. Artichoke treats liver and gall bladder disorders, as well as irritable bowel syndrome and nausea. It's also valuable as a diuretic, helping to relieve water retention and high blood pressure. The youth-enhancing antioxidant flavonoids found in artichokes help to keep the arteries healthy.

NUTRIENTS
Vitamins B3, B5, C, biotin, folic acid; cynarin; iron, potassium, zinc

---

HOT ARTICHOKE DIP WITH PITTA BREAD

8 pitta breads
225g/8oz cream cheese
350g/12oz mozzarella
200g/7oz/1 cup mayonnaise
150g/5½oz/1 cup grated
   Parmesan
1 onion, finely chopped
2 cloves garlic, crushed
375g/13oz/2½ cups marinated
   artichoke hearts

Preheat the oven to 350°F/ 180°C/Gas mark 4. Cut the pitta breads into small triangles, and bake on a tray. Combine the other ingredients in a food processor and blend. Put mixture in a dish, and cook in the oven for 30 minutes. Serve hot with the pitta dippers.

sweet potato

Containing vitamins C and E, sweet potatoes are a fantastic youth-preserving food.

NUTRIENTS
Vitamins B6, C, E, beta-carotene; iron, potassium; fibre

Sweet potatoes are extremely rich in antioxidants. They are one of the few foods containing both vitamins C and E, which work synergistically with one another to help to stave off wrinkles, and to preserve the eyes and the memory. Orange sweet potatoes are abundant in beta-carotene, which keeps the skin, eyes and lungs healthy, and supports the immune system, along with vitamin C. They also contain vitamin B6, which preserves memory and protects the heart.

HERBY SWEET POTATO WEDGES

6 medium sweet potatoes
handful each of fresh oregano
  and thyme sprigs
olive oil
freshly ground black pepper

Preheat the oven to 350°F/ 180°C/Gas mark 4. Scrub the sweet potatoes and cut them lengthways into chunky, wedge-shaped pieces. Put them in a baking dish. Break up the herbs and place them with the olive oil and black pepper with the sweet potatoes. Toss well. Bake for about 30 minutes until soft.

040

radish

Part of the Cruciferae family, radishes contain many nutrients to fight premature ageing.

Radishes are rich in sulphur, which is essential for youthful, healthy skin, hair and nails, and also has anti-carcinogenic properties. Assisting the body in ridding itself of toxins, radishes help to treat gall bladder and liver problems, which might cause premature ageing. They are also a valuable source of potassium to keep the heart healthy, calcium to help prevent osteoporosis, vitamin C to fight against eye problems and selenium to boost immunity.

NUTRIENTS
Vitamin C, folic acid; calcium, potassium, selenium, sulphur

RADISH SLAW

200g/7oz radishes, trimmed and coarsely grated
300g/10½oz green cabbage, finely shredded
1 large carrot, coarsely grated
1 small red onion
2 tbsp fresh lemon juice
½ tsp sugar
2 tbsp extra virgin olive oil
handful of fresh coriander
salt and pepper, to taste

Combine all the ingredients in a bowl and mix well. Store in the fridge and use within 2 days.

mushroom

NUTRIENTS
Vitamins B12, E; phosphorus, potassium, selenium; protein

Mushrooms have more protein than most vegetables, as well as vitamin E and selenium.

A rich source of anti-ageing vitamin E and selenium, mushrooms help to maintain healthy skin and hair, and protect against heart disease. They also boost immunity and have anti-carcinogenic properties. Mushrooms contain potassium, which is central to heart health, and vitamin B12, which holds off arthritis. Shiitake mushrooms specifically boost immunity, while the reishi variety combat high blood pressure and asthma, and maitake treat blood pressure and liver disease.

GLAZED SHIITAKE MUSHROOMS

450g/1lb shiitake mushrooms
1 tsp rapeseed oil
80ml/2½fl oz/⅓ cup chicken stock
1 tsp cornflour
2 tsp soy sauce
1 tbsp dry sherry

Wash the mushrooms, discard the stems and slice. In a large saucepan heat the oil and add the mushrooms and 2 tablespoonfuls of the stock. Cook, stirring often, for 5–6 minutes. In a small bowl dissolve the cornflour in the remaining stock. Stir in the soy sauce and sherry; add to the pan. Cook for 2 minutes, or until the mushrooms are glazed.

asparagus

A renowned aphrodisiac, asparagus contains Vitamin E to keep the skin and the heart youthful.

Asparagus is a fantastic source of folic acid, which is said to prevent damage to the arteries that supply blood to the heart and the brain. Folic acid has also demonstrated anti-carcinogenic properties. Asparagus contains asparagine, which, along with its high potassium and low sodium content, makes it an excellent diuretic and cleanser. The vegetable is also high in vitamin E to fight wrinkles, protect the heart and keep the brain young.

NUTRIENTS
Vitamins B3, C, beta-carotene, folic acid; potassium, zinc; asparagin; flavonoids; fibre

BALSAMIC ROASTED ASPARAGUS

500g/1lb 2oz large asparagus spears, trimmed
2 tbsp extra virgin olive oil
sea salt and freshly ground pepper
2 tbsp balsamic vinegar
finely grated lemon rind, for garnish

Preheat the oven to 400°F/200°C/ Gas mark 6. Coat the asparagus spears in the olive oil and season with salt and pepper. Roast on foil on a baking tray for 20–25 minutes, turning them 2–3 times. Drizzle with balsamic vinegar. Garnish with lemon rind.

043

◐ ◉ ♥ ✚

Brussels sprout

NUTRIENTS
B-vitamins, vitamin C, folic acid;
phytonutrients; fibre

Full of plant compounds, B-vitamins, vitamin C and fibre, Brussels sprouts help to keep us free from many conditions associated with ageing.

Brussels sprouts are crammed with phytonutrients, such as sulforaphane, which triggers the release of detoxifying and anti-carcinogenic enzymes. The vegetables are also rich in fibre, thus staving off digestive complaints. Brussels sprouts have lots of immunity-building vitamin C, which keeps us youthful by preventing eye disease and protecting the memory. They are also a source of folic acid, which fights heart disease.

BRUSSELS SPROUTS WITH BACON

**450g/1lb Brussels sprouts,
trimmed and washed
115g/4oz back bacon, diced
100g/3½oz/¼ cup roasted,
salted pistachios, shelled
60ml/2fl oz/¼ cup balsamic
vinegar**

Steam the Brussels sprouts for 5–10 minutes, until almost tender. In a frying pan cook the bacon until crisp. Remove, and add the Brussels sprouts to the pan; sauté for 1–2 minutes. Add the pistachios and vinegar. Continue to cook for 1–2 minutes, reducing the vinegar and glazing the sprouts and nuts. Add the bacon, season, mix well and serve.

Swiss chard

Rich in iron and other health-giving nutrients, Swiss chard is important for any anti-ageing diet.

The iron in Swiss chard helps the body to produce red blood cells to transport oxygen. Swiss chard also contains vitamin C, which improves iron absorption in the body, as well helping to eliminate toxic heavy metals and prevent hair loss. The high levels of B-vitamins and minerals such as magnesium, potassium and calcium protect the heart, while its carotenoid content fights cell damage by free radicals.

NUTRIENTS
B-vitamins, vitamin C, carotenoids; calcium, iron, magnesium, potassium, selenium

CREAMED SWISS CHARD

1 tbsp olive oil
1 medium onion, sliced
450g/1lb Swiss chard
1 tbsp plain flour
250ml/9fl oz/1 cup evaporated skimmed milk
2 tsp grated Parmesan
pinch of ground nutmeg

In a heavy saucepan, heat the oil. Add the onion, and cook for 5–6 minutes on a low heat. Chop the chard into ribbons, and add to the pan. Cover and cook for a further 3–4 minutes. Sprinkle in the flour and add the milk, stirring continuously, until the sauce thickens. Add the Parmesan and the nutmeg. Mix well and serve.

bok choy

NUTRIENTS:
Vitamins A, C; calcium

The freshest bok choy has firm white stalks and dark green leaves.

Popular in Chinese cooking, bok choy has a light, sweet flavour and is high in vitamins A and C, and calcium.

A type of Chinese cabbage, bok choy is unique in that it's one of the few vegetables to contain high levels of vitamin A, which is especially useful for maintaining eye health. It's also rich in antioxidant vitamin C, helping to keep youthful everything from the immune system to the gums, and the heart to the skin. Bok choy contains plenty of calcium for bones and teeth. It's also low in sodium and in calories, thus is a good choice for weight control.

BABY BOK CHOY IN SZECHWAN SAUCE

8 baby bok choy, quartered lengthways
2 tbsp peanut oil
2 tsp grated ginger
½ tsp red chilli paste
1 tbsp hoisin sauce

In a wok stir-fry the bok choy in the oil for about 3 minutes. Add the ginger and stir-fry for a further 2 minutes. Then, add the chilli paste and hoisin sauce, and stir-fry for a further minute. Serve immediately.

carrot

With their very high levels of beta-carotene, carrots have powerful anti-ageing properties.

Beta-carotene, which the body converts into vitamin A, is especially important for eye health. It's also of great benefit to the skin, and the immune and digestive systems. Along with alpha-carotene, it is anti-carcinogenic and helps to reduce the risk of heart disease. Carrots are also loaded with fibre and water, which cleanse the liver, boost detoxification and plump out the skin to stave off wrinkles. The vitamin C and silica content of carrots is also valuable for keeping the skin youthful.

Because carrot tops leach out the carrots' nutrients, cut them off before storing.

NUTRIENTS
Vitamins C, K, alpha-carotene, beta-carotene, folic acid; calcium, iron, silica, zinc; fibre

BEAUTY JUICE
(for skin, hair and nails)

4 cucumbers
4 parsnips
8–12 carrots, scrubbed,
    with tops removed
2 lemons, peeled
1 green pepper

Cut the cucumber and parsnip lengthways and feed through a juicer, followed by the carrots, lemons and green pepper. Pour into glasses and serve.

pumpkin

NUTRIENTS
Vitamin C, carotenoids; fibre

Pumpkin has high levels of carotenoids and antioxidants to stave off premature ageing.

Bright orange in colour, pumpkins are high in carotenoids, including beta-carotene, which have anti-carcinogenic properties and prevent heart disease and eye problems. Beta-carotene also helps to protect against the harmful and ageing effects of the sun. Pumpkin contains plenty of vitamin C, which boosts immunity and preserves the skin.

PUMPKIN, PARSNIP AND CARROT SOUP

1 tbsp extra virgin olive oil
15g/½oz butter
1 onion, chopped
250g/8oz pumpkin, skinned and deseeded
250g/8oz parsnips
250g/8oz carrots
900ml/34fl oz/3½ cups chicken or vegetable stock
1–2 tbsp lemon juice

Chop the vegetables. Heat the oil and butter in a saucepan and fry the onion until soft. Add the pumpkin, parsnips and carrots, and stir well. Cover, and cook gently for 5 minutes. Add the stock. Bring to the boil, cover and simmer for 30 minutes. Leave to cool, then blend until smooth. Reheat in the pan and add lemon juice to taste. Serve.

048

Brazil nut

Brazil nuts are high in "good" fats and are full of selenium, which keeps us young and healthy.

Brazil nuts are about 70 per cent fat. Half of this is oleic acid, the building block for the omega-9 fatty acids that are excellent for the skin and have anti-inflammatory properties. The rest is made up of omega-6 and omega-3 essential fatty acids, which promote healthy skin, glossy hair and a good memory. The abundant levels of vitamin E and selenium provide a strong boost to the immune system, while selenium also activates glutathione, which destroys harmful free radicals.

NUTRIENTS
Vitamin E; calcium, magnesium, selenium; oleic acid, omega-3 and omega-6 fatty acids; fibre; protein

BRAZIL NUT PESTO

handful of flat leaf parsley, coarsely chopped
80g/2¾oz Brazil nuts, coarsely chopped
1½ tbsp water
pinch of tarragon, chopped
1 clove garlic, crushed
½ tsp grated lemon rind
3 tbsp extra virgin olive oil
2 tbsp Parmesan, grated
salt and pepper to taste

Preheat the oven to 400°F/ 200°C/Gas mark 6. In a food processor combine the parsley, Brazil nuts, water, tarragon, garlic and lemon rind into a coarse paste. Add the olive oil and the Parmesan, and blend until smooth. Serve.

almond

NUTRIENTS

B-vitamins, vitamin E, essential fatty acids; iron, magnesium, potassium, zinc; plant sterols; protein; fibre

To enhance the flavour of almonds, toast them in a pan over low heat until golden.

Almonds contain a host of oils and nutrients that are especially good for keeping the skin youthful.

Almonds are a good source of protein, needed for healthy growth and the repair of cells. The nuts also contain more fibre than any other nut, thereby helping to maintain good digestion. Their calcium content helps to keep bones strong and to stave off osteoporosis. They also contain monounsaturated fats and plant sterols, which help to reduce the risk of heart disease.

VITAMIN E FOR RADIANT SKIN

Almonds are a fantastic source of vitamin E, which plays an important role in maintaining healthy skin both internally and

ALMOND AND OATMEAL HOTCAKES

60g/2¼oz/⅓ cup plain flour
155g 5½oz/⅔ cup oatmeal
2 tsp baking powder
30g/1oz ground almonds
1 egg
250ml/9fl oz/1 cup soya milk
cooking oil

Mix the flour, oatmeal, baking powder and almonds together in a bowl. In a separate bowl, lightly beat the egg and soya milk and add to the dry ingredients; mix well. Put a splash of oil in a shallow pan, heat well, and add about

125ml/4fl oz of the mixture. When golden and bubbles form on the upper side, turn and cook the other side. Repeat with the remaining mixture to make several hotcakes. Serve with bananas, honey and yoghurt.

externally, helping to preserve elasticity and repair damage. Almond oil, especially, is wonderfully soothing for the skin and effective in healing post-operative scars. Vitamin E also boosts immunity and protects the heart.

ABUNDANT MINERALS

Almonds provide zinc, magnesium and potassium. While zinc strengthens immunity, magnesium increases energy and potassium reduces blood pressure, staving off heart disease.

TRADITIONAL ALMOND MILK *(to nourish the skin)*

50g/1¾oz ground almonds
2 tbsp honey
500ml/17fl oz/2 cups still
mineral water

In a bowl combine the almonds, honey and water. Stir well, until the honey has dissolved. Leave for 2 hours. Filter, and pour into a bottle with a lid. Apply generously to the face and neck with cotton wool, and leave on for 20 minutes. Use in the morning and evening. Keeps for up to 3 days in the fridge.

walnut

NUTRIENTS
B-vitamins, vitamin E; copper, magnesium, potassium, zinc; omega-3 fatty acids; protein

Walnuts are a wonderful snack food, providing many nutrients as well as a healthy oil.

Walnuts and walnut oil contain protein, vitamins B6 and E, potassium, magnesium, copper and zinc, all of which help to keep us youthful. Vitamin B6 helps to prevent memory loss and protect the heart, while vitamin E maintains skin and hair. Both potassium and magnesium are good for the heart, and copper helps to prevent varicose veins. Zinc has a miraculous ability to rejuvenate the thymus gland and to boost immunity. Walnut oil is a good source of fatty acids, central to skin and heart health.

WALNUT, APPLE AND CELERY STUFFING

85g/3oz/⅓ cup butter
1 large onion, finely chopped
2 stalks celery, finely chopped
2 cooking apples, chopped
350g/12oz breadcrumbs
225g/8oz chopped walnuts
½ tsp dried thyme
1 large egg, beaten
125ml/4fl oz/½ cup milk

Preheat oven to 350°F/180°C/ Gas mark 4. Cook the butter, onion and celery in a saucepan. Mix the apples, breadcrumbs, walnuts and thyme in a bowl; stir in the vegetables, egg and milk. Spoon into a baking dish. Bake for 30 minutes. Serve.

cashew nut

Seeds of the Brazilian "cashew apple", cashew nuts are full of healthy fats and protein.

Cashew nuts are a great source of omega-6 essential fatty acids, which protect against heart disease. The nuts also contain magnesium, a nutrient that aids the function of the heart and enables the metabolism of calcium, which prevents osteoporosis. Rich in B-vitamins, which aid the maintenance of nerves and muscle tissue, and boost resistance to stress, cashews contain selenium to stave off wrinkles and promote glossy hair. They also provide iron to help to prevent anaemia.

NUTRIENTS
B-vitamins, biotin, folic acid; iron, magnesium, manganese, potassium, selenium, zinc; omega-6 fatty acids; iodine; protein; fibre

CASHEW NUT CREAM

110g/4oz cashew nuts
100ml/4fl oz/½ cup soya milk
1 tsp runny honey
100ml/4fl oz sunflower oil
1 tsp lemon juice

Put the cashew nuts and soya milk in a blender and blend until creamy. Add the honey, and slowly pour in the oil – you will notice the mixture thicken – then, add the lemon juice to set the cream. Serve chilled. Keeps in the fridge for up to 5 days.

peanut

Peanuts are full of heart-healthy nutrients and provide the most protein of all nuts.

NUTRIENTS
Vitamin E, folic acid; potassium; arginine; fibre

Peanuts are high in monounsaturated fats, which reduce cholesterol levels and protect against clogged arteries and heart disease. The heart is protected further by the amino acid arginine, which the body converts to nitric oxide, helping to expand blood vessels and prevent clotting. Peanuts are also high in vitamin E, which maintains wrinkle-free skin and glossy hair. Because of their low glycaemic index score, the nuts also help to prevent adult-onset diabetes.

SPICY CHICKEN SATAY

100g/3½oz roasted peanuts,
  coarsely chopped
2 garlic cloves, crushed
½ tsp ground ginger
1 tsp curry powder
1 tsp ground coriander
60ml/2fl oz/¼ cup soy sauce
2 tbsp sesame oil
1 tbsp brown sugar
pinch of chilli powder
3 chicken breasts, skinless,
  chunked and put on skewers

In a frying pan cook the peanuts, garlic and ginger for 2 minutes, then add all the other ingredients. Leave to marinate overnight. Preheat the oven to 325°F/165°C/Gas mark 3. Place the skewers of chicken in a dish. Pour the marinade over and bake for 10 minutes.

sesame seed

These tiny, nutrient-rich seeds were a symbol of immortality in ancient India.

Youth-enhancing sesame seeds and their oil are good sources of vitamin E, plus omega-6 and monounsaturated fats, which help to minimize heart disease and maintain healthy skin and hair. They also contain B-vitamins to support the nervous system and to help the body to cope with stress. The seeds and oil are an excellent source of calcium and magnesium, which are necessary for bone and heart health. They are rich in zinc to boost immunity, as well as selenium to stave off wrinkles.

NUTRIENTS
B-vitamins, vitamin E: calcium, iron, magnesium, zinc; omega-6 and omega-9 fatty acids

SESAME TAHINI DIP

350g/12oz/1¼ cups sesame seeds
4 tbsp peanut oil

Preheat the oven to 350°F/ 180°C/ Gas mark 4. Sprinkle the sesame seeds on to a baking sheet and toast in the oven for 20 minutes. Whizz the seeds in a blender for about 3 minutes, then add 1 tablespoonful of oil and whizz for 30 seconds before adding the remaining oil. Whizz again until a smooth paste is formed. Serve with roasted vegetable pieces.

sunflower seed

Although small, sunflower seeds are powerhouses of youth-enhancing antioxidant nutrients.

Sunflower seeds and oil are full of vitamin E, omega-6 essential fatty acids and monounsaturated fats, which help to keep the skin elastic and minimize heart disease. Omega-6 also helps to fight inflammation, thus relieving arthritis. The seeds and oil are rich in calcium and magnesium, needed for the contraction of muscles as well as a healthy bone structure. Magnesium is also used in producing energy. Sunflower seeds and oil also contain immunity-boosting zinc and selenium.

NUTRIENTS

B-vitamins, vitamin E; calcium, copper, magnesium, manganese, selenium, zinc; omega-6 fatty acids; protein

---

SUNFLOWER SEED OAT BREAD *(makes 2 small loaves)*

500g/1lb 2oz oat flour/ 5 cups
6g/¼ oz instant dried yeast
2 tbsp sunflower seeds
1 tsp salt
2 tbsp malt extract
400ml/14fl oz/⅔ pint warm water
1 tbsp sunflower oil

Preheat the oven to 350°F/ 180°C/Gas mark 4. Put the flour, yeast, seeds, salt and malt extract in a bowl; mix well. Add the water and oil. Form a dough. Knead for 10 minutes; divide into 2 and place in loaf tins. Cover and leave for 30 minutes. Bake for 50–60 minutes until browned.

O 🐾 🍥 ♡ 😺 ✚ ◐

pumpkin seed

Tasty and nutritious, pumpkin seeds are full of essential fatty acids and micronutrients.

The abundant essential fatty acids found in pumpkin seeds are vital for youthful skin and glossy hair. EFAs are also central to a healthy brain, to boosting immune function and decreasing inflammation. Pumpkin seeds are particularly high in zinc, offering defence against infections and boosting fertility. Together, EFAs and zinc have been linked to reducing prostate problems. Pumpkin seeds also contain calcium and magnesium for healthy bones, nerves and muscles.

NUTRIENTS
B-vitamins; calcium, magnesium, selenium, zinc; omega-3 and omega-6 fatty acids; protein

PUMPKIN SEED BRITTLE

60g/2¼oz/⅓ cup sugar
60ml/2fl oz/¼ cup water
100g/3½ oz/½ cup pumpkin
  seeds, toasted
1tsp extra virgin olive oil
pinch of salt

Toss the pumpkin seeds in a bowl with the oil and a pinch of salt. Then, spread them evenly on a baking sheet in the middle of a preheated oven at 250°F/ 120°C/Gas mark ½ for an hour; stir occasionally. In a frying pan combine the sugar and water, stirring continuously over low heat, until a deep caramel colour. Add the seeds, and stir until well coated. Turn out on to a greased sheet of foil. Let cool completely and break into pieces.

flaxseed

NUTRIENTS
Calcium, magnesium, zinc; omega-3 and omega-6 fatty acids; lignans

With a sweet, nutty taste, flaxseeds are loaded with essential fats for a youthful body and brain.

Flaxseeds and flaxseed oil are full of omega-3 and omega-6 essential fatty acids, which are central to youthful-looking skin and hair, an alert mind, a healthy heart and an efficient immune system. The seeds and the oil also contain lignans, which have anti-carcenogenic properties. In addition, they provide calcium and magnesium for healthy bones.

To make flaxseeds more digestible, soak them in water for a few hours before eating them.

FLAXSEED FACE MASK
(to smoothe wrinkles)

2 tsp flaxseeds
water, enough to cover
1 drop neroli oil

In a small bowl, combine the flaxseeds and water. Leave to stand until the seeds swell and the water turns to gel, then add the neroli oil. Using your fingers, spread the gel over your face and neck. Allow to dry then rinse off with cool or tepid water. Pat your face dry.

057

oats

Oats are very versatile and are useful for preventing heart disease and boosting immunity.

As well as being a good source of energy-giving carbohydrates, oats are high in fibre, therefore maintaining steady blood sugar levels and preventing diabetes, and lowering cholesterol. They contain powerful, youth-promoting antioxidants, including vitamin E, tocotrienol, ferulic acid and caffeic acid to fight against free radicals and protect against everything from heart disease to obesity and eye disease. Used topically, oats have a soothing, anti-inflammatory effect on the skin.

NUTRIENTS
B-vitamins, vitamin E, folic acid; iron, magnesium, selenium, silica, zinc; saponins; tocotrienol, ferulic acid, caffeic acid; protein; fibre

OATMEAL HERBAL SCRUB
(to decongest the skin)

3 tbsp dried parsley, lemon balm or fennel seeds
160ml/5¼fl oz/⅔ cup boiling water
1 tbsp ground oatmeal
2 drops almond oil

Make a herbal infusion by pouring the water over the herbs and covering for 15 minutes. Strain and discard the herbs. Allow the infusion to cool, then add enough to the oatmeal to form a paste-like consistency. Add the almond oil. Smooth the scrub on the face and neck and leave for 20 minutes. Then, rinse off with tepid water and pat dry.

barley

NUTRIENTS
B-vitamins, vitamin E; selenium;
tocotrienol; lignans; fibre

A great grain for the heart, barley is also full of antioxidants to fight damaging free radicals and the effects of ageing.

Barley is the oldest cultivated cereal, and it was used widely by the Romans as a strengthening food. Today, it is largely neglected, but it has amazing nutritional properties.

BARLEY LOTION
(to improve blood circulation)

100g/3½oz pearl barley
1 litre/35fl oz/4 cups water
generous handful of fresh
**   rosemary or 3 tbsp dried**
**   rosemary**

Cover the barley with cold water and soak for 24 hours. Drain, and put the barley in a saucepan with the fresh water. Bring to the boil, cover and simmer for 30 minutes. Strain and discard the barley. Add the rosemary to the barley water, cover and leave to infuse until cool. Strain into a secure glass bottle. Using cotton wool, apply twice daily. Store in the fridge for up to 4 days.

A HEALTHY HEART

Barley is one of the richest sources of the antioxidant tocotrienol, which studies have shown to be even more potent than some forms of vitamin E in preventing heart disease. It works in two ways. First, they help to stop free radical oxidation, a process that makes "bad" cholesterol more likely to stick to artery walls. And second, they act on the liver to reduce cholesterol production. The grain also contains lignans that help to prevent tiny blood clots from forming, further reducing the risk of heart disease.

VALUABLE NUTRIENTS

Barley is exceptionally high in both selenium and vitamin E, which together have anti-carcinogenic properties. Vitamin E plays a pivotal role in keeping the skin and hair healthy and young-looking, while selenium is efective in fighting viral infections, protecting the heart from muscle damage and the eyes from disease.

Barley also contains calcium, potassium and B-vitamins, which help to keep the bones strong, blood pressure in check and the nervous system and the brain healthy. In addition, barley is full of soluble fibre, which aids digestion.

Pot barley is better than pearl barley, as it retains much more fibre.

whole wheat

NUTRIENTS
Vitamins B6, E; magnesium, zinc; pyroxidine; protein; fibre

A staple food in the Western diet, wheat is protein-rich, providing B-vitamins and minerals.

Whole wheat is a nutritious and healthy cereal grain. A valuable source of protein, it provides the building blocks for youthful skin, hair and nails. It also provides a valuable source of energy, thus combating fatigue. Whole wheat is rich in B-vitamins, including B6, which maintains the nerves, prevents adult-onset diabetes and also enhances the ability to register, retain and retrieve information. The grain is a good source of zinc, which boosts immunity and aids eye health.

SIMPLE WHOLEWHEAT PIZZA CRUST

540g/1lb 3oz/4 cups whole wheat flour
2 tbsp active dry yeast
1½ tsp salt
500ml/17fl oz/2 cups warm water
2 tbsp extra virgin olive oil
2 tsp honey
topping of choice

Preheat the oven to 400°F/ 200°C/ Gas mark 6. Combine the flour, yeast and salt in a bowl. Add the water, oil and honey; mix well. Cover with a moist cloth and leave to rise in a warm place for 10 minutes. Knead and press into a greased large pizza pan. Add the topping. Then, bake for 15–20 minutes.

brown rice

Brown rice is an excellent source of fibre, as well as many valuable youth-preserving nutrients.

Fibre-rich brown rice keeps the digestive system in good health and helps to lower cholesterol in the blood. It's very high in B-vitamins, which are needed for a healthy brain and nervous system. Brown rice is also a source of magnesium, easing high blood pressure and helping the body to turn food into energy and prevent muscle cramps. Containing iron to combat anaemia and premature hair loss, brown rice is also high in zinc, which promotes good immunity and healthy eyes. It is also said to boost sexual vigour.

NUTRIENTS
B-vitamins, folic acid; copper, iron, magnesium, manganese, zinc; protein; fibre

BROWN RICE PUDDING

1 litre/35fl oz/4 cups water
300g/10½oz/1½ cups brown short-grain rice
600ml/21fl oz/2½ cups soya milk
4 tbsp rice or date syrup
1 tsp ground cinnamon
¼ nutmeg, grated
4 whole cloves
2 small handfuls of raisins
4 shavings of orange rind

Preheat the oven to 350°F/ 180°C/Gas mark 4. Put the water ina saucepan; bring to the boil. Add the rice and simmer for 15 minutes. Strain and return the rice to the pan. Add the remaining ingredients and simmer for 20 minutes. Turn into a lightly greased dish. Bake for 40 minutes.

millet

Extremely easy to digest, millet is particularly high in silica, which helps to keep the skin youthful.

NUTRIENTS
Magnesium, potassium, silica; protein

MILLET PILAFF

1 large onion, finely chopped
4 tsp extra virgin olive oil
2 tbsp ground coriander seeds
2 cloves garlic, crushed
250g/9oz/2 cups millet
600g/1lb 5oz tomatoes
600ml/21fl oz/2½ cups
    vegetable stock
250ml/9fl oz/1 cup white wine
2 tsp flaked almonds
4–5 dashes of soy sauce

Preheat the oven to 350°F/ 180°C Gas mark 4. Gently fry the onion in oil for 4–5 minutes. Add the coriander and garlic; fry for 5 minutes. Add the millet and cook for 2 minutes. Add the tomatoes, stock and wine. Boil, then simmer uncovered for 20 minutes, until tender. Add the almonds and soy sauce. Serve.

A fantastic source of silica, millet is a central ingredient in collagen, the body's "glue", which is needed for healthy hair, skin, teeth, eyes, nails, tendons and bones. Silica also prevents cardiovascular disease and plays an important role in memory function. Besides being easily digestible, millet is the only alkaline-forming grain, thus helping to counteract over-acidity in the stomach and joints. It is also protein-rich, containing all eight essential amino acids that aid recovery after illness.

quinoa

Quinoa provides a spectrum of B-vitamins for health and youthfulness.

A complete protein, quinoa helps tissue to grow and also repairs it. Quinoa contains several B-vitamins, including B5, which is essential for a healthy response to stress. Full of iron, it is a high-energy grain, thus preventing fatigue, as well as hair loss and anaemia. It also supplies the body with magnesium, which is well-known for preventing high blood pressure, and vitamin B2, which controls cholesterol build-up by destroying harmful free radicals. Quinoa also contains vitamin E, which is good for the skin.

NUTRIENTS
B-vitamins, vitamin E; calcium, iron, magnesium, zinc; saponins; protein; fibre

QUINOA TABBOULEH

200g/7oz/1 cup quinoa
400ml/14fl oz/ 1¾ cups
   vegetable broth
2 tbsp pine nuts, toasted
8 cherry tomatoes, finely
   chopped
2 onions, finely chopped
1 tbsp each parsley, mint and
   coriander, finely chopped
4 tbsp fresh lemon juice
2 tbsp extra virgin olive oil

Rinse and drain the quinoa, then put in a saucepan. Toast for 3 minutes. Add the broth and bring to the boil. Reduce heat, cover and simmer for 12 minutes. Drain and put in a bowl. Add the pine nuts, tomatoes, onions and herbs. In a dish combine the lemon juice and olive oil, and pour over the salad. Mix well and serve.

063

buckwheat

NUTRIENTS
B-vitamins, magnesium, rutin; protein; fibre

Buckwheat is high in rutin, a substance that strengthens tiny blood vessels.

Because of its rutin content, buckwheat is associated with circulatory health – it strengthens blood capillaries, thus preventing the formation of thread veins. Buckwheat contains fibre and all eight essential amino acids, and is a good source of protein for the brain. Rich in magnesium, the grain contains B-vitamins, which help to maintain the nervous system. It also lowers blood cholesterol levels.

BUCKWHEAT MUESLI

200g/7oz/2½ cups buckwheat flakes
100g/3½oz/⅓ cup oats
50g/1¾oz/½ cup sunflower seeds
50g/1¾oz/1 cup dried apricots
50g/1¾oz/⅓ cup raisins

Chop the apricots into bite-size pieces. In a large mixing bowl, combine the ingredients thoroughly. The muesli keeps well in a sealed plastic container. Serve with milk or soya milk.

lentil

A staple food in many countries, lentils are one of the single most nutritious and digestible foods.

Whether red, green or brown, lentils are a great source of protein, which we need to keep our skin, hair, teeth and nails strong and healthy. Lentils also contain high levels of B-vitamins, particularly B3, which protects against poor memory, and B12, which helps to prevent everything from arthritis to tinnitus. Lentils are rich in iron, thus preventing anaemia. They are also full of fibre and help to regulate digestion.

NUTRIENTS
B-vitamins, folic acid; calcium, iron, potassium, selenium, zinc; protein; fibre

LENTIL AND CUMIN SOUP

2 onions, roughly chopped
4 cloves garlic, crushed
4 tsp cumin seeds
3 tbsp vegetable oil
1 bay leaf
½ tsp dried oregano
3 litres/104fl oz/12 cups chicken stock
600g/1lb 5oz/3 cups tinned green or brown lentils

In a saucepan sauté the onion, garlic and cumin seeds in the oil. Add the bay leaf, oregano and stock. Bring to the boil and simmer for 10 minutes. Add the lentils and cook for a further 10 minutes. Remove the bay leaf and purée the soup in a food processor. Serve garnished with sour cream and toasted cumin seeds.

soya bean

NUTRIENTS
B-vitamins, vitamin E, folic acid; calcium, magnesium, manganese, potassium, zinc; phytic acid; saponins, isoflavones

---

SCRAMBLED TOFU

2 cloves garlic, crushed
½ large red pepper, diced
2 tbsp extra virgin olive oil
300g/10½oz firm tofu
½ tsp turmeric
½ tsp salt
pinch of black pepper
1 medium onion, chopped
1½ tsp soy sauce

In a frying pan sauté the garlic and pepper in the olive oil for 2 minutes. Crumble the tofu and add to the pan, then add the turmeric, salt, pepper, onions and soy sauce. Cook for 3 minutes, stirring occasionally. Remove from the heat. Serve with salsa and corn tortillas.

Eating a diet rich in soya beans is believed to help to prevent heart disease, as well as to promote youthfulness and longevity.

This versatile legume is central to the diet of the Japanese, who have the longest life spans in the world. In Western countries, soya is best known in its derivative forms – as tofu, soya milk, soya yoghurt, soy sauce and as meat analogues, for example textured vegetable protein (TVP).

FIGHTING DEGENERATIVE DISEASES

Soya beans are an excellent source of plant protein, dietary fibre and complex carbohydrates. They are known to have a cholesterol-lowering effect and to prevent high triglyceride levels, which can cause heart disease. In addition, soya beans contain youth-preserving antioxidants, such as phytic acid, which can help to prevent clogging of the arteries.

However, perhaps the most useful attribute of soya beans is that they are extremely rich in micronutrients, such as saponins and isoflavones. A type of flavonoid, isoflavones are converted by the body into phytoestrogens and have anti-carcinogenic properties as well as the ability to promote bone health and reduce the risk of cardiovascular disease.

The beans contain vitamin E, which is vital for preserving youthful skin and hair, and B-vitamins, which maintain the nervous system and keep stress from causing premature ageing. The beans also have an extremely low glycaemic index score, thus helping to prevent diabetes and alleviating various menopausal symptoms.

When buying soya products, it is worth taking the time to check that they are free from GM soya.

chickpea

NUTRIENTS
B-vitamins, vitamin E, folic acid;
iron, potassium, zinc; protein; fibre

Chickpeas have a unique savoury, nutty flavour
and are rich in many youth-preserving nutrients.

Chickpeas are a good source of protein, which is vital for the
healthy repair of cells. Their high vitamin E content boosts the
immune system, protects the heart and promotes healthy skin
and hair. They also contain zinc, which enhances immunity
and rejuvenates the thymus gland. In addition, chickpeas are a
useful source of isoflavones, which mimic oestrogen and have
anti-carcenogenic properties.

BAKED CHILLI CHICKPEAS

3 onions, sliced
1 fresh chilli pepper, finely
**   chopped**
150ml/5fl oz/⅔ cup extra
**   virgin olive oil**
4 cloves garlic
2 tbsp dried oregano
550g/1 lb 3½oz/3 cups tinned
**   chickpeas**

Preheat the oven to 300°F/
150°C/Gas mark 2. Sauté the
onions and chilli pepper in the
oil until soft, then add the
garlic, oregano and chickpeas;
mix well and transfer to an
oven-proof dish. Add enough
water to cover the chickpeas,
put lid on and bake for 1–1½
hours or until tender. Add more
water during cooking if needed.

067

kidney bean

Kidney beans are high in protein, fibre and nutrients that maintain health and well-being.

Popular in Central and South America, kidney beans are an excellent source of protein, which helps to keep energy levels steady as well as maintaining cells. They are also rich in folic acid, which is good for healing wounds, and to help prevent heart disease. Kidney beans are full of fibre, which is vital for keeping cholesterol levels down and aiding digestion. They are also a valuable source of iron, helping to prevent anaemia.

NUTRIENTS
Folic acid; iron, manganese, potassium, protein, fibre

KIDNEY BEAN GUMBO

1 red onion, chopped
1 red pepper, deseeded and
   diced
1 stalk celery, chopped
2 cloves garlic, crushed
1 tbsp olive oil
1.5 litres/52fl oz/6 cups
   vegetable stock
425g/15oz/1½ cups diced
   tomatoes
1 tsp dried thyme
pinch of cayenne pepper
270g/9½ oz/1½ cups tinned
   kidney beans

In a saucepan fry the onion, pepper, celery and garlic in the oil for 5 minutes. Add the stock, tomatoes, thyme and cayenne; cover and simmer until soft. Add the kidney beans and simmer for 10 minutes. Serve.

sardine

Fresh and tinned sardines contain a host of age-defying fatty acids and antioxidants.

Some of the most beneficial nutrients for keeping our skin looking young and radiant are omega-3 fatty acids, and sardines are an excellent source.

PROTECT THE SKIN

However, the benefits of omega-3 fats are more than skin-deep. Several studies show that they help to make the blood less liable to clot and so reduce the risk of heart disease. They also keep the eyes healthy. In addition, research suggests that they

GRILLED SARDINES WITH SALSA VERDE

2 large onions, chopped
2 cloves garlic, peeled
2 large green peppers, deseeded and chopped
125ml/4fl oz/½ cup extra virgin olive oil
50g/2oz tinned anchovies
2 small green chillis, deseeded

zest and juice of 2 lemons
2 tbsp capers
8 tbsp chopped basil
4 level tbsp chopped parsley
12 fresh sardines, washed

In a saucepan gently heat the onion, garlic and peppers with half

the oil. Put in a food processor with the anchovies, chillies, lemon zest and juice, capers and herbs and whizz into a chunky purée. Grill the sardines on foil under a hot grill for 5–7 minutes on each side. Lay on a plate, drizzle over the salsa and serve.

may help to protect the skin against sun exposure and ultra-violet radiation.

ANTIOXIDANT-RICH

Sardines also provide selenium, a powerful antioxidant that helps to prevent wrinkles and heart disease. Selenium is anti-carcinogenic and neutralizes toxic metals in the body.

Tinned sardines are a good source of calcium, which keeps bones strong and healthy.

690

salmon

Wild salmon is full of omega-3 fatty acids, which are renowned for their anti-ageing properties.

Salmon is one of nature's best sources of omega-3 fatty acids as well as DHA (docosahexaenoic acid), both of which are renowned for reducing cardiovascular disease. They are also good for keeping the skin and hair youthful. Essential fatty acids have powerful anti-inflammatory properties, making them useful for arthritic conditions. DHA is especially important for the brain and the nervous system, helping to keep the memory working well.

NUTRIENTS

Vitamins A, B12, D; omega-3 fatty acids, dimethylaminoethenol, docosahexaenoic acid

WATERCRESS SALMON STEAKS

4 salmon steaks
4 tsp extra virgin olive oil
juice of 1 lemon
bunch of watercress, washed
  and chopped
4 tbsp mayonnaise
1 tsp Tabasco sauce (optional)

Put the salmon steaks on a grill pan. Drizzle 1 teaspoonful of olive oil and lemon over each. Grill each side under medium heat for 5 minutes. Put the watercress, mayonnaise and remaining lemon juice in a blender and whizz until smooth. Season with salt, pepper and Tabasco (if using). Spoon over the salmon and serve.

prawn

Prawns are an excellent source of B-vitamins and minerals with youth-enhancing attributes.

Prawns are rich in vitamin B12, which promotes brain function and prevents fatigue, and vitamin B3, which is crucial for preserving the memory. Their selenium content is anti-carcinogenic and essential for heart health. Selenium also fights off wrinkles. Prawns supply iodine, which is vital for the proper functioning of the thyroid gland, and calcium for strong bones. They are also rich in zinc, which boosts immunity and fertility.

NUTRIENTS
B-vitamins; calcium, iodine, magnesium, phosphorus, potassium, selenium, zinc; protein

PRAWN PÂTÉ

450g/1lb prawns, shelled and cooked
3 tbsp butter
3 tbsp cream cheese
1 tbsp sour cream
2 drops Tabasco sauce
½ tsp ground nutmeg
I clove garlic, crushed
1 tbsp lemon juice
pinch of salt and pepper

Put the prawns (reserving one) in a blender with all the other ingredients. Whizz until smooth. Place the pâté in a serving dish and garnish with the whole prawn. Serve with hot toast triangles.

herring

NUTRIENTS

B-vitamins, vitamin, A, D, E; omega-3 essential fatty acids; protein

With up to 20 per cent of their weight being made up of essential fatty acids, herring are an important anti-ageing food.

High in omega-3 fats, herring has extremely powerful anti-inflammatory properties, thus preventing and relieving arthritic conditions, reducing the risk of cardiovascular disease and protecting the memory. Herring is high in zinc, which boosts the immune system. It is a protein-rich food and also contains many vitamins – the fat-soluble vitamins A, D and E, as well as the water-soluble B-vitamins.

When buying kippers (smoked herring), choose undyed fish to avoid added chemicals.

PICKLED HERRING

185ml/6fl oz/¾ cup water
185ml/6fl oz/¾ cup white vinegar
2 cloves garlic
¼ tsp dill seeds
80g/2¾oz granulated sugar
900g/2lb salt herring fillets
1 red onion, sliced into rings

In a saucepan bring the water, vinegar, seasonings and sugar to the boil, stirring until the sugar dissolves. Leave to cool. Cut the herring into 2.4cm/1in pieces, removing the bones. In 2 large jars, arrange the herring and the onion rings in alternate layers. Cover with the pickling solution. Chill for at least 3 days before serving. Store for up to 3 weeks.

haddock

A member of the cod family, haddock contains many nutrients to help us stay younger and fitter.

Haddock contains several B-vitamins to boost brain power and fight fatigue. It's especially high in folic acid, which helps to protect against heart disease, diabetes and osteoporosis by reducing the body's levels of homocysteine. Folic acid may also have anti-carcinogenic properties. Haddock is an excellent source of iodine, which is needed to produce thyroid hormones that regulate the body's metabolism. The fish also contains zinc for immunity, sulphur to beautify the skin, and calcium to boost bone health and help to prevent conditions such as osteoporosis.

NUTRIENTS
B-vitamins, folic acid; calcium, iodine, sulphur, zinc; essential fatty acids protein

BEER BATTERED HADDOCK

125g/4½oz/1 cup flour
pinch of salt and pepper
275ml/9fl oz/1 bottle beer
900g/2lb fresh haddock

In a bowl, combine the flour, salt, pepper and beer. Cut the haddock into pieces and dip into the batter. Then put them directly in a saucepan of hot oil. Cook on a low to medium heat for 5 minutes on each side or until golden.

oyster

NUTRIENTS
Vitamins B3, B12, D, E; calcium, iron, magnesium, selenium, zinc

A renowned aphrodisiac, oysters are packed with health-boosting vitamins and minerals.

Oysters contain vitamins B3 and B12, which are useful to prevent memory problems. They are a valuable source of zinc, which helps to build resistance to disease, maintain youthful skin and prevent hair loss. Oysters also contain vitamin E, which is also good for the skin and for preventing heart disease, as well as conditions such as arthritis. The shellfish are an excellent source of iron, which combats anaemia. They provide vitamin D, as well, for healthy bones and teeth.

OYSTER BISQUE

2 pints/4 cups oysters, shelled
450ml/16fl oz/1 pint vegetable stock
salt
white pepper
900ml/32fl oz/4 cups milk
225ml/8fl oz/1 cup cream
1 tbsp potato flour
a little butter

In a saucepan boil the oysters in the stock for about 30 minutes. Strain, then add the salt, pepper, milk and cream. Simmer gently for 2 minutes. Mix the potato flour with the butter; add to the saucepan and stir to thicken. Serve.

lamb

Lean lamb is an excellent source of protein and easily absorbed iron.

NUTRIENTS
B-vitamins; iron, selenium, sulphur; protein

High in protein, which is necessary for the repair of ageing cells, lamb is also a rich source of B-vitamins, including vitamin B12, which is vital for a healthy heart. The meat is also high in easily absorbed iron, which is fundamental for preventing anaemia. The selenium in lamb protects the eyes from disease and the heart from muscle damage. Lamb is a source of sulphur, good for strong hair and nails.

Some lamb contains growth hormones, so always opt for organic, free-range lamb.

LAMB SHANKS IN TOMATO-ORANGE SAUCE

4 lamb shanks
450g/1lb crushed tomatoes
250ml/9fl oz/1 cup water
1 tbsp crushed garlic
rind and juice of 1 orange
2 tbsp fresh mint, finely chopped

Lightly grease a large saucepan. Add the lamb and cook, turning as needed, for 10 minutes or until lightly browned on all sides. Add the tomatoes, water, garlic, orange rind and juice to the pan. Cover and simmer for 2–3 hours or until the meat is tender. Stir in the mint, and serve.

beef

Beef contains many nutrients, especially iron, which boosts the oxygen level in the blood.

A good source of protein, beef is also high in B-vitamins, including B12, which prevents fatigue and memory loss. It is rich in iron, which staves off conditions such as anaemia and premature hair loss. Free-range, grass-fed beef is a good source of conjugated linoleic acid (CLA), a fatty acid shown to promote weight loss. Beef is also a source of sulphur, which our bodies need to maintain youthful hair and nails.

BEEF STIR-FRY

4 tbsp soy sauce
2 tbsp dark roasted sesame oil
900g/2lb beef steak, cut into strips
4 cloves garlic
2 tbsp minced fresh ginger
¼ tsp chilli flakes
2 red peppers, sliced

Combine the soy sauce and half the oil and pour over the beef. Heat the remaining oil, add the garlic, ginger and chilli flakes and cook for 30 seconds. Stir-fry the pepper for 2 minutes. Remove from the pan, add the beef and cook over high heat for 3–4 minutes. Add the vegetables and reheat.

chicken

Extremely popular and hugely versatile, chicken is bursting with health-giving nutrients.

Chicken is a good source of protein, contributing to the growth and repair of the body's cells, and, with the skin removed, is low in fat. It's rich in selenium, which helps to prevent wrinkles and keep the hair glossy. Chicken also contains iron and zinc to boost energy levels and immunity – there is twice as much in the dark meat as in the breast. The breast is particularly high in vitamin B6, which protects the heart.

NUTRIENTS
Vitamins B3, B6; iron, potassium, selenium, zinc; protein

SWEET AND SOUR CHICKEN DRUMSTICKS

8 chicken drumsticks, skinned
4 tbsp runny honey
2 tbsp sesame oil
90ml/3fl oz/⅓ cup soy sauce
4 tsbp lemon juice
4 tsp coarsegrain mustard

Preheat the oven to 200°C/400°F/Gas mark 6. Put the drumsticks in an ovenproof dish and pierce with a fork. Mix the honey, sesame oil, soy sauce, lemon juice and mustard and pour over the chicken. Cook for 25–30 minutes. Serve hot or cold.

eggs

NUTRIENTS:
Vitamins A, B, D, E, lutein; selenium, zinc; lecithin, choline, zeaxanthin; protein

Eggs, both the whites and yolks, pack a powerful punch when it comes to anti-ageing nutrients.

Protein- rich, eggs contain all eight essential amino acids, thus helping to make up the building blocks for the entire body – benefiting everything from skin to hair, and bones to muscles.

LOADED WITH VITAMINS

Eggs are also a wonderful source of zinc and vitamins A, B, D and E. The zinc helps to boost immunity and is also vital for the production of collagen, which is needed for healthy, youthful skin. Vitamin A supports vision, vitamin D promotes strong bones and vitamin E benefits the heart. Eggs are also a valuable source of selenium, which rejuvenates the immune system and protects the heart.

BRAIN FOOD

Owing to their high lecithin content, eggs are an important brain food, contributing not only to memory and concentration, but also to a healthy emotional state. Egg yolk is the richest known source of choline, which makes up cell membranes, helping the body to convert fats to acetylcholine, an important memory molecule in the brain.

EGG YOLK MASK
(to nourish dry skin)

1 tbsp honey
1 large egg yolk
1 tsp potato flour

In a bowl combine the honey, egg yolk and potato flour, stirring to create a fine paste. Apply evenly to the face and neck and leave for about 20 minutes. Rinse off with cotton wool and water. Pat dry. Repeat 2 or 3 times a week, making a fresh mask for each treatment.

CHOLESTEROL CONCERN

Many of us worry about the apparently high cholesterol content of eggs, but studies suggest this may be unfounded as the cholesterol in eggs doesn't circulate in the blood. In fact, of the 5g of fat contained in an egg, most is monounsaturated, which is the type that helps to lower the risk of heart disease.

Egg whites, as well as yolks, can be used in face masks, as they have great astringent qualities.

078

milk

NUTRIENTS: Vitamins B12, E; calcium, potassium

Best known for its calcium content, milk helps to strengthen the bones and fight off heart disease.

The abundance of calcium in milk gives it the ability to strengthen bones and to help to stave off osteoporosis. Studies have also shown that calcium may help to reduce blood pressure as well as cholesterol levels. Milk is a good source of vitamin B12, which combats memory and hearing problems, and fatigue. It also contains vitamin E, which benefits the eyes, skin and immune system. Its potassium content is key in fighting heart disease. Skimmed milk is also believed to have anti-carcinogenic properties.

> Even if you don't like to drink milk, you can add it to recipes to increase your intake.

MINT MILK BATH *(to nourish the skin and protect from ageing)*

125g/4½oz/1 cup cornstarch
250g/9oz/2 cups dried milk powder
4 tsp crushed mint leaves
100g/3½oz/½ cup sea salt

Put all the ingredients in a jar and shake well to combine them. Add about 125g/4½ oz/ 1 cup to running bath water. To obtain maximum benefit, soak in the bath for 15 minutes.

bio-yoghurt

Made by adding "friendly" bacteria to milk,
bio-yoghurt fights ageing, both inside and out.

The live bacteria lactobacillus and bifidobacteria found in
bio-yoghurt help to maintain the correct level of acidity in
the gut, and also enhance immunity. In addition, they lower
cholesterol levels, reducing the risk of heart disease. Yoghurt is
rich in protein and calcium, which are essential for healthy
bones and efficient muscles and nerves. Its vitamin B content
boosts energy and protects the nervous system.

NUTRIENTS:
Vitamins A, B, C; calcium, iron,
phosphorus, potassium, sodium;
protein

**BIO-YOGHURT AND
LEMON CLEANSER**

**2 tsp bio-yoghurt
1 tbsp lemon juice**

Mix the ingredients together
in a small bowl. Apply to the
face and neck area, and leave
for 10 minutes. Rinse off with
warm water and pat dry. (As
well as acting as a cleansing
agent, the bio-yoghurt will
have a cooling and refreshing
action on your skin, while also
rebalancing your skin's pH
value. The yoghurt's lactic
acid content will brighten your
skin, too.).

green tea

GREEN TEA AND PEACH REFRESHER

2 ripe peaches, stoned and sliced
1.5 litres/52fl oz/6 cups cold water
6 green tea teabags
honey, to taste
sprigs of mint

Put the peaches in a saucepan, add the water and bring to the boil. Put the teabags in a large pitcher and pour the water and peaches over them. Steep for 6 minutes, then add the honey to taste. Allow to cool, then refrigerate until chilled. Pour the tea and peach slices into glasses and garnish with mint to serve.

Extremely high in bioflavonoids, green tea neutralizes the damaging effects of free radicals and fights premature ageing.

Tea is the most popular beverage in the world, and green tea (comprising leaves that are lightly steamed when cut, rather than left to dry out like black tea) is fast becoming recognized for its youth-enhancing properties.

TREATS CONDITIONS

Green tea contains phenolic compounds that help to strengthen blood vessels, which makes it useful for treating conditions such as thread or varicose veins, as well as cold hands or feet. It also contains good amounts of vitamin E to help to boost immunity, promote healthy, glowing skin and protect the eyes and the heart. The tannins in green tea offer further benefits for the eyes, as they act as an anti-inflammatory to relieve puffiness.

AMAZING ANTIOXIDANTS

The antioxidant bioflavonoids in green tea offer fantastic protection against heart and circulatory problems and have anti-carcinogenic properties. They also help to ward off wrinkles and preserve eye health. Bioflavonoids are said to rev up the metabolism and promote weight loss.

HEART HEALTHY

Green tea is also said to lower "bad" LDL cholesterol and triglyceride levels and raise "good" HDL cholesterol levels.

When making a cup of green tea, steep it for at least 3 minutes to gain its full benefits.

081

garlic

NUTRIENTS
Vitamin B6, C; calcium, sulphur; s-allylcysteine

Part of the onion family, garlic is famous for its anti-viral and heart-protecting properties.

Garlic contains a sulphur compound called allicin, which is released when garlic is crushed, encouraging the elimination of cholesterol from the body, lowering triglyceride levels, detoxifying the liver and acting as a potent anti-inflammatory. Its sulphur means that garlic helps in the formation of new cells, keeping the skin, nails and hair young-looking. It is also said to help to treat cellulite. Garlic contains a compound, called s-allylcysteine, which appears to have an anti-carcinogenic action. Garlic is also a powerful immunity booster.

GARLIC BATH SOAK
(to soothe arthritis)

1 large fresh bulb garlic

Crush the garlic and add it to running bath water. Relax and soak in the bath for at least 15 minutes to gain the full anti-inflammatory benefits.

082

parsley

Parsley is full of youth-enhancing nutrients and is a natural healer.

Parsley is the richest herbal source of the mineral potassium, which reduces high blood pressure – the number one cause of heart attacks. Potassium also stimulates the kidneys to eliminate waste matter. Parsley has anti-inflammatory properties, thus protecting against arthritis. It's also an excellent source of vitamin A for the eyes, and magnesium and calcium to protect the bones and the nervous system. The herb is rich in manganese, which boosts the memory, iron to prevent fatigue and vitamin C for strong immunity.

NUTRIENTS
Vitamins A, B, C; calcium, copper, iron, magnesium, potassium

Potassium is destroyed in cooking, so eat parsley raw to obtain maximum benefits.

FRESH PARSLEY MASK
(to tone and nourish the skin)

1 tbsp chopped parsley
1 tbsp honey
1 tbsp fresh milk

In a bowl combine all the ingredients and mix into a thin paste. Apply to the face and leave for 20 minutes. Rinse off with warm water and pat dry.

ginger

NUTRIENTS
Vitamin B6; potassium, magnesium, copper, manganese; gingerol

Ginger boosts the digestive system and has excellent anti-inflammatory properties.

Ginger protects the digestive system against premature ageing, thus aiding the general absorption of nutrients. The root helps to regulate blood sugar, both by stimulating pancreas cells and by lowering cholesterol levels. Because ginger is such an effective anti-inflammatory, it is among the most respected herbs for the treatment of joint problems such as arthritis. Its main active constituent is gingerol, which has strong antioxidant properties. Ginger also boosts blood circulation.

GINGER BEER

2 litres/ 70fl oz bottle still
   mineral water
250g/9oz/1 cup sugar
plastic funnel
¼ tsp dried yeast
juice of 1 lemon
1½–2 tbsp grated ginger root

Decant the bottled water into another container. Pour the sugar into the empty bottle through the funnel, then add the yeast. Mix the lemon juice with the ginger. Using the funnel, pour the mixture into the bottle. Add the water (leaving a 2.5cm/1in gap at the top). Shake well and leave in a warm place for 24–48 hours, then store in the fridge overnight. Pour into glasses through a strainer. Serve.

084

turmeric

With its bright yellow colour, turmeric offers a range of youth-enhancing benefits.

Turmeric is perhaps best known for its ability to relieve inflammatory conditions. It contains curcumin, a potent antioxidant, which is very effective at fighting free radicals and therefore protects the skin, eyes and hair, and keeps them youthful. Curcumin also has anti-bacterial, anti-carcinogenic and cholesterol-lowering properties. It is an anti-coagulant, therefore reducing the risk of heart attacks. Research shows that curcumin may also protect against memory deterioration.

NUTRIENTS
Vitamins A, C; curcumin; iron

Avoid exposure to the sun if taking turmeric medicinally, as it can increase sensitivity.

SEA BASS WITH TURMERIC AND LIME RUB

1 tsp salt
juice of 1 lime
1 tsp turmeric powder
4 sea bass fillets
3 tbsp vegetable oil

In a bowl, mix the salt, lime juice and turmeric together. Rub into the sea bass fillets. Heat the oil in a non-stick frying pan, add the coated fillets and cook for 2–3 minutes on each side. Serve with a vegetable dhal.

fennel

NUTRIENTS
Vitamin C, folic acid; potassium; phytonutrients; fibre

Especially popular in French and Italian cuisine, fennel boasts a host of anti-ageing properties.

Rich in phytonutrients, including rutin, quercetin and anethole – the primary components of its volatile oil – fennel has been shown to reduce inflammatory conditions such as arthritis. It is also an excellent source of vitamin C, which is needed for the proper functioning of the immune system, to protect the brain and to avoid ageing of the arteries. Fennel is fibre-rich and may help to reduce elevated cholesterol levels. In addition, it's a good source of folic acid, a vitamin that lowers the risk of heart disease.

FENNEL SEED INFUSION *(to cleanse and tone the skin)*

2 tsp fennel seeds, crushed
2 sprigs fresh thyme, crumbled,
or ½ tsp dried thyme
125ml/4fl oz/½ cup boiling water
juice of ½ a lemon

In a bowl, combine the fennel seeds and thyme, and cover with the boiling water. Add the lemon juice and steep for 15 minutes. Strain, and when cold, store, covered, in a jar in the fridge. Dab evenly on the face and neck every morning with cotton wool, then rinse off with warm water.

086

dandelion

Dandelion aids detoxification, thus keeping the body free of age-accelerating toxins.

With its detoxifying action dandelion is useful for treating water retention, promoting weight loss and boosting energy. It's also a good source of beta-carotene and lutein, which have anti-carcinogenic properties. Dandelion contains vital nutrients including vitamins A, B and C. Vitamin A keeps the eyes young and healthy, while B-vitamins maintain the nervous system and the brain. Vitamin C is key to immune function and also protects the heart. Dandelion is high in calcium for the bones, and copper, which helps to prevent varicose veins.

NUTRIENTS
Vitamin A, B, C, D; calcium, copper, iron, potassium

DANDELION AND MANDARIN SALAD

3 tbsp extra virgin olive oil
3 tsp cider vinegar or lemon juice
140g/5oz dandelion leaves
150g/5½oz/¾ cup sliced spring onions
6 hard-boiled eggs, sliced
200g/7oz/1½ cups mandarin segments
dandelion flowers (optional)

Combine the oil and vinegar to make the dressing. In a salad bowl, combine the dandelion leaves and onions; add the dressing and toss to coat. Arrange on 4 plates; top with the eggs and mandarin segments. Garnish with dandelion flowers if desired.

cayenne pepper

NUTRIENTS
Vitamins A, B, C; calcium, manganese, potassium; capsaicin; fibre

Hot and spicy, cayenne pepper is packed with nutrients to keep the symptoms of ageing at bay.

Cayenne pepper is a rich source of vitamins A and C, as well as all the B-vitamins. It's therefore useful for everything from eye health to immune function, and healthy skin to good memory. Cayenne is also very high in calcium, which staves off osteoporosis, and potassium, which is good for the heart. The pepper has a high concentration of capsaicin, which has been widely studied for its pain-reducing effects, cardiovascular benefits and ability to help to prevent ulcers. Capsaicin also gives cayenne its anti-inflammatory properties.

WARMING CAYENNE WAX
(to treat painful, inflamed joints)

225g/8oz beeswax
2 fresh cayenne peppers,
 or 1 dried cayenne pepper
3ml/⅗ tsp St John's Wort

In a saucepan melt the beeswax and add the cayenne pepper. Simmer for 10 minutes, then remove the pepper. Stir in the St John's Wort. Pour the warm mixture into empty ice cube trays and freeze. Melt 1 cube as needed. As it melts, lay out some tissue and, using a pastry brush, paint on the wax in a strip. Wrap the tissue strip around the painful area. To retain heat, cover the area in cling film. Leave on for 20 minutes. Repeat 3 times a week.

chamomile

Best known as a relaxant, chamomile is a popular remedy for insomnia and digestive complaints.

Chamomile relaxes the muscles throughout the body. Its bitters stimulate the flow of bile and the secretion of digestive juices, enhancing the appetite and improving sluggish digestion. The herb is very soothing and helps to induce relaxation and sleep. Used topically, chamomile treats inflamed joints and stiff muscles. It also has cosmetic benefits: when used in face creams, it promotes a youthful, glowing complexion. Chamomile is also known for being a powerful conditioner that leaves the hair softer and shinier.

NUTRIENTS
Flavonoids; tannins

CHAMOMILE HAIR TREATMENT

handful of chamomile flowers
80ml/2½fl oz/⅓ cup olive oil

Combine the chamomile and oil in a jar with a lid. Stand on a sunny windowsill and shake at least once a day. After 2 weeks, strain and discard the chamomile. Brush out your hair and apply to the hair ends, avoiding the scalp, using about 2–4 teaspoonfuls, depending on the length of your hair. Leave on for about 10 minutes, then shampoo as normal.

⬤ ♥ ✚ ⦿

ginseng

NUTRIENTS
Choline; saponins

The Chinese have revered ginseng for 5,000 years as an overall antidote to the ravages of ageing.

Ginseng is a renowned performance enhancer, not just for physical work but for mental tasks, too. A great energizer, ginseng helps to combat fatigue and is also believed to fight heart disease, as well as combat impotence. Ginseng contains choline, a chemical vital to the brain for learning and memory retention. It also contains antioxidants to defy the effects of ageing, and compounds with oestrogenic properties, which relieve menopausal symptoms.

SPICED GINSENG ICED TEA

2 litres/70fl oz/8 cups water
8 cardamom pods, crushed
6 whole cloves
2 cinnamon sticks
1 star anise pod
8 ginseng teabags
60ml/2fl oz/¼ cup honey
ice cubes

In a large saucepan combine the water with the cardamom pods, cloves, cinnamon sticks and star anise, and bring to the boil. Remove from the heat and add the teabags; allow them to steep for 5 minutes. Remove the teabags and stir in the honey until dissolved. Strain the tea into a jug and leave to cool, then refrigerate until chilled. Serve in tall glasses over ice.

paprika

Commonly found in powdered form, paprika is a wonderful circulatory stimulant.

Paprika derives its bright, orange-red colour from carotenoid pigments, which protect the body from free-radical damage. The spice also has a high concentration of capsaicin, recognized for its pain-reducing effects, as well as its cardiovascular benefits. Capsaicin's anti-inflammatory properties make paprika useful for the treatment of arthritis. Paprika also contains sizeable amounts of vitamin C, which is vital for youthful skin and a strong immune system.

NUTRIENTS
B-vitamins, Vitamin C, carotenoids; capsaicin; anthocyanins

BAKED COD WITH PAPRIKA

2 or 3 onions, sliced
1 tsp paprika
60g/2¼oz/¼ cup butter
1.3 kg/3lb cod fillets, skinned
juice of 1 lemon
salt and pepper
pinch of dried rosemary
125ml/4fl oz/½ cup sour cream

Preheat the oven to 375°F/ 190°C/Gas mark 5. Sauté the onions, with half the paprika in half the butter. Mix the lemon juice with water in a bowl and rinse the cod. Put in a baking dish with remaining butter. Season with salt, pepper, rosemary and rest of paprika. Cover with onions and sour cream. Bake for 30 minutes.

gingko biloba

An extract from the gingko leaf, gingko biloba has a remarkable ability to improve memory.

NUTRIENTS
Flavonoids

GINGKO BILOBA AND ROSEMARY TONIC

handful of dried gingko leaves
handful of dried rosemary
enough vodka to cover

Place the gingko in a jar, cover with vodka and secure the lid. Repeat the process with the rosemary in a separate jar. Every few days shake the jars vigorously. After 4 weeks, strain the mixtures and discard the herbs. Combine the tinctures in 1 bottle. Put ½–1 teaspoonful of the tincture in a cup of hot water, stir and leave for a few minutes (this will allow most of the alcohol to evaporate). Take the tonic 2–3 times a day, preferably on an empty stomach.

As we become older, our bodies typically produce fewer neurotransmitters, and our brain tends to be more forgetful and less alert. However, gingko biloba is said to increase the production of dopamine, which improves the brain's ability to transmit information. Research has also demonstrated that gingko improves the blood circulation, thus helping the brain and other organs to function efficiently. Gingko is rich in flavonoids, which are anti-carcinogenic and help to protect the body from heart disease and arthritis.

wheatgrass

Positively bursting with nutrients, wheatgrass is an elixir of youthfulness.

Wheatgrass contains all the vitamins except vitamin D. It's also rich in enzymes, minerals and proteins. This makes it good for everything from the nervous system to the circulatory system, to eye health and skin elasticity. Wheatgrass is said to help to prevent tooth decay, and to stop hair going grey. Its high chlorophyll content boosts production of blood. Wheatgrass also helps to combat the toxins in the body, which left unchecked, can accelerate the ageing process.

NUTRIENTS
Vitamin A, B-vitamins, vitamins C, E, K; calcium, magnesium, manganese, phosphorus, potassium, selenium, zinc; chlorophyll

GREEN GARDEN COCKTAIL

1 tray fresh wheatgrass
2 sticks celery
handful of parsley
masticating juicer

To harvest the wheatgrass, grasp a small bundle of blades firmly, and with a sharp knife, cut them off above the compost level. Rinse all the ingredients in cold water and feed them into a masticating juicer. Repeat with 2–3 more bundles of wheatgrass. Drink about 2 tablespoonfuls/each day on an empty stomach.

water

LEMON AND MINT WAKE-UP WATER

1 lemon
handful of mint leaves
500ml/17fl oz/2 cups water

Slice the lemon and place in a large pitcher. Carefully rub the mint leaves between the palms of your hands to bruise them slightly. Add them to the pitcher. Pour in the water, cover and chill overnight. In the morning strain the water mixture and discard the mint. Return the lemon slices to the water, pour into a large glass and sip.

Water is essential to our health and survival, and is well known for its revitalizing properties.

Water is central to our well-being. This is perhaps not surprising, given that the average adult is made up of about 70 per cent water. However, most of us don't drink enough of it, and as a result, we live in a constant state of dehydration.

VITAL TO THE BODY

If our bodies don't have sufficient water, they can't eliminate waste products effectively, which causes problems such as kidney stones. Water is vital for the blood circulation and for chemical reactions in the digestive and metabolic processes. It carries nutrients and oxygen to cells through the blood, thus stimulating the organs. It also lubricates our joints, keeping us supple and agile. We need water for energy, and even to breathe – our lungs must be moist to take in oxygen. And, perhaps surprisingly, we also require plenty of water to avoid water retention and excess weight gain.

SKIN SAVIOUR

Water also regulates and controls the natural pH balance of the skin – revitalizing, hydrating, oxygenating and detoxifying it. Without water, the body is unable to rid itself of the harmful toxins that get trapped in the tissues, causing the complexion to deteriorate. Water is also needed to keep hair shiny and healthy.

WATER THERAPY
(to regulate the skin's natural pH balance)

A shower!

Adjust the water so that the temperature is comfortably hot, and shower for 1 minute. Then, adjust the temperature to cold, and shower for another minute. Repeat, alternating between hot and cold bursts for another 5 minutes, or longer. Finish with a blast of cold water. Step out of the shower, wrap yourself in a warm towel and relax for a while before dressing.

alfalfa sprout

Alfalfa sprouts are highly digestible and contain huge amounts of antioxidants.

These sprouted seeds provide abundant amounts of vitamin A for the eyes, B-vitamins for the nervous system and brain power, vitamin C for immunity and eye health, and vitamin E for the skin and the heart. They are also high in calcium and phosphorus for the bones, iron to prevent anaemia, magnesium and potassium to lower the risk of heart disease, zinc to prevent premature hair loss, and silica to promote glowing skin, strong nails and glossy hair.

NUTRIENTS

Vitamin A, B-vitamins, vitamins C, E; calcium, magnesium, phosphorus, potassium, silica, zinc; chlorophyll

SUNSHINE PITTA POCKETS

1 cauliflower, steamed
¼ tsp dry mustard
juice of ½ a lemon
½ tsp curry powder
tiny pinch of salt
¼ tsp ground cardamom
70g/2½oz/⅓ cup mayonnaise
4 pitta breads
115g/4oz alfalfa sprouts
3 carrots, grated
2 tomatoes, sliced

Mash the cauliflower in a bowl and mix in the mustard, lemon juice, curry powder, salt, cardamom and mayonnaise. Chill in the fridge. Halve the pitta breads, divide the mixture between them, then add the sprouts, carrots and tomatoes.

095

wheatgerm

The sprouting part of wheat grain, wheatgerm is a super source of free-radical-fighting vitamin E.

Owing to its high vitamin E content, wheatgerm is especially good for keeping hair glossy and skin glowing. It's also been shown to prevent heart disease. Wheatgerm contains omega-6 fatty acids, thus relieving pain in the joints. Its choline content produces the neurotransmitter acetylcholine, which helps to boost memory. The brain also benefits from its B-vitamins. Used topically, wheatgerm's slightly granular texture gently exfoliates sensitive or dry skin.

NUTRIENTS
B-vitamins, vitamin E; iron, magnesium, manganese, selenium, zinc; omega-6 fatty acids; choline; fibre

WHEATGERM EXFOLIATING LOTION

250ml/9fl oz/1 cup milk
85g/3oz/1 cup dried
   chamomile
4 tbsp honey
8 tsp wheatgerm

Pour the milk into a cup and add the chamomile. Leave to infuse for a few hours. Strain the liquid and discard the chamomile. Add the honey and wheatgerm, and mix well. Pour the lotion into a bottle and store in the fridge for up to a week. Apply to the face and neck, then rinse off with warm water. Use as needed.

brewers yeast

NUTRIENTS
B-vitamins; magnesium, zinc; lecithin, lipoic acid; protein

Brewers yeast is especially useful to boost energy levels and brain power.

Comprising almost 50 per cent protein, as well as some lecithin and unrivalled levels of B-vitamins, brewers yeast is a valuable remedy for fatigue and lapses of memory. It's also rich in lipoic acid, which helps to keep the brain young and active. Brewers yeast is a good source of zinc to boost the immune system, as well as magnesium to promote a healthy heart. Used topically it is very effective for treating dry skin complaints. Holding up to 70 per cent moisture, it provides the building blocks for regenerating soft, supple and healthy tissue.

BREWERS YEAST FACE PACK

**1 tsp crushed fennel seeds
125ml/4fl oz/½ cup water1
tbsp brewers yeast**

In a small saucepan, simmer the fennel seeds in the water for 10 minutes, then strain. Allow the infusion to cool to room temperature, then mix in the brewers yeast. Spread the mixture over the face and neck, and leave for 10 minutes. Rinse off gently with warm water and pat dry.

097

cider vinegar

Made from fermented apple juice, cider vinegar is well known for its anti-arthritic properties.

The malic acid content of apple cider vinegar helps to dissolve calcium deposits in the body and eases arthritis. It also helps to balance the body's acid-alkaline pH levels and oxygenates the blood, thus aiding digestion and boosting the immune system. Enzyme-rich, cider vinegar contains the perfect balance of 19 minerals, as well as apple pectin, the water-soluble dietary fibre that binds to toxins in the body and assists in their removal, thus improving skin tone. Pectin also lowers cholesterol levels, and so helps to stave off heart disease.

NUTRIENTS
Iron, calcium, chlorine, fluorine, magnesium, potassium, phosphorus, silica, sodium, sulphur; malic acid; fibre

Apple cider vinegar is available as a fibre supplement, and is said to help with weight loss.

CIDER VINEGAR HAIR RINSE *(to restore dull, lifeless hair)*

1–2 tbsp apple cider vinegar
750ml/26fl oz/3 cups water

Mix the cider vinegar and water in a jug. After shampooing and conditioning your hair as usual, pour the cider vinegar mixture over your hair as a final rinse.

honey

NUTRIENTS
B-vitamins; calcium, copper,
iron, magnesium, manganese,
phosphorus, potassium, sodium,
zinc

FIRMING FACE MASK

1 tbsp honey
1 egg white
1 tsp glycerin
about 30g/1oz/¼ cup flour

In a small bowl, mix the honey,
egg white and glycerin. Then,
add enough flour to form a
paste. Smooth the mask over
the face and throat. Leave for
10 minutes, then rinse off
gently with warm water.

Best known as an energy food, honey also has
many anti-ageing properties.

Widely used as a natural sweetener, honey is composed of
79 per cent sugar. The rest comprises water and small amounts
of vitamins, including vitamin B6, which is good for the brain,
and many minerals, including calcium to strengthen the
bones. Honey also contains phytonutrients such as propolis,
which helps to boost immunity, and caffeic acid, which has
anti-carcinogenic properties. Used topically, honey is a
humectant, attracting and retaining water, which keeps the skin
soft and supple.

coconut oil

Coconut oil is a unique source of medium-chain fatty acids – a great aid to staying youthful.

Coconut oil is extremely rich in medium-chain fatty acids (MCFAs), which are soluble and a great energy source, similar to carbohydrates. MCFAs have been shown to assist the absorption of calcium, magnesium and some amino acids, as well as supporting the healthy function of the thyroid. MCFAs, particularly lauric acid, are great immunity boosters. They also stimulate metabolism, benefit the heart and promote weight loss. Rich in vitamin E, coconut oil keeps the skin's connective tissues strong and supple, which helps to prevent wrinkles.

NUTRIENTS
Vitamin E; medium-chain fatty acids

COCONUT BODY OIL

80ml/2½fl oz tub of coconut oil
15 drops of your favourite essential oil

Remove the lid from the coconut oil and place the tub in a large saucepan with water; heat gently, until the oil liquefies. Add your favourite essential oil and stir well. Replace the lid back and put the tub in the fridge for 15 minutes. Apply generously all over your body (but not to your face). Beware that the oil could stain your clothes, so avoid dressing until the oil has soaked well into the skin.

olive oil

NUTRIENTS
Vitamin E; oleic acid; polyphenols; monounsaturated fats

A Mediterranean favourite, olive oil contains fats and antioxidants that are central to good health and youthful beauty.

Made from the crushing and the subsequent pressing of olives, olive oil contains vitamin E, which helps to keep skin wrinkle-free and hair glossy.

Always choose extra virgin olive oil, as this contains the optimum nutrients.

HOT OIL TREATMENT
(to treat a dry scalp and hair)

125ml/4fl oz/½ cup olive oil
125ml/4fl oz/½ cup boiling water

Pour the olive oil and boiling water into a large glass bottle or a jar with a lid. Shake well until the oil is emulsified. When the mixture has cooled slightly, massage into the hair, taking care not to burn the scalp. Put a shower cap or plastic bag over your hair and wrap it in a hot towel that has been soaked in hot water, then wrung out. Leave for about 30 minutes, then shampoo as usual.

GOOD FATS

Olive oil is also rich in monounsaturated fat, which is believed to have anti-carcinogenic properties, and help to lower high blood pressure and prevent diabetes.

HEART HEALTHY

Research into the effectiveness of olive oil against clogging of the arteries reveals that the olives' monounsaturated fats prevent the oxidation of cholesterol, and therefore stop it from sticking to artery walls and causing heart attacks. Further studies suggest that olive oil also contains hefty concentrations of antioxidants, including chlorophyll, carotenoids and polyphenolic compounds – all of which not only fight age-accelerating free radicals, but also protect the olives' important vitamin E content. Their rich supply of polyphenols, known to have anti-inflammatory and anticoagulant actions, are also thought to help stave off conditions such as osteoporosis and arthritis.

BEAUTIFUL SKIN

Olive oil is high in oleic acid, an omega-9 fatty acid, which demonstrates anti-inflammatory properties to calm and soothe the skin.

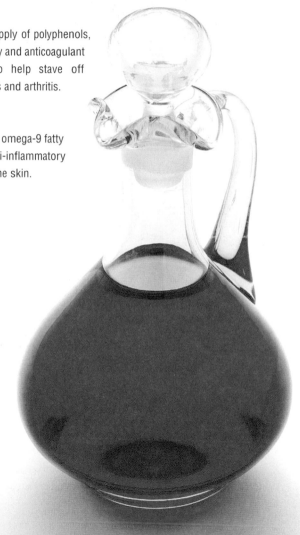

OLIVE OIL AND LEMON
DRINK *(to soothe inflammation)*

2 tbsp extra virgin olive oil
juice of ½ lemon

In a cup combine the olive oil and the lemon juice. Mix well. Drink on an empty stomach every morning and wait for at least 30 minutes before having breakfast. Repeat for at least 3 weeks to notice an improvement.

ailments directory

WRINKLES

We can get wrinkles at any age from our 20s onwards, depending on our life style and our genetic predisposition. Factors such as smoking, spending lots of time in the sun and using sunbeds can all age the skin prematurely and exacerbate lines, particularly around the eyes. To fight wrinkles, reduce sun damage and improve skin texture, eat foods full of vitamins A, C and E, and selenium.

Foods to eat:

Grape (p.10); Avocado (p.34); Onion (p.41); Radish (p.51); Almond (p.60); Cashew nut (p.63); Sesame seed (p.65); Chicken (p.91); Green tea (p.96)

LACKLUSTRE HAIR

As we age, our hair follicles slowly become dormant – a natural process in both men and women. However, foods rich in iron and vitamin A nourish the hair follicles and can help to keep your hair looking thick and lustrous.

Foods to eat:

Prune (p.20); Spinach (p.45); Watercress (p.48); Swiss chard (p.55); Almond (p.60); Prawn (p.85); Beef (p.90)

FATIGUE

If you feel tired all the time, you could well be anaemic. This condition occurs when there is a decrease in the amount of oxygen-carrying haemoglobin found in your red blood cells. Symptoms include weakness, pale skin and general fatigue. Eating foods rich in iron and vitamin B12 help to combat anaemia at any stage in life.

Foods to eat:

Spinach (p.45); Almond (p.60); Cashew nut (p.63); Quinoa (p.75); Lentil (p.77); Kidney bean (p.81); sardine (p.82) Lamb (p.89); Beef (p.90)

INSOMNIA

Sleep quality is a key factor in how you look and feel – good sleep makes you perform better both mentally and physically, and helps your eyes, skin and hair to stay healthy and bright. To get a good night's sleep, avoid stimulants such as coffee and chocolate for at least 5 hours before you go to bed, as they can interrupt sleep patterns or cause blood sugar highs and lows. Also, when snacking, eat foods containing natural sugars to keep your blood sugar levels stable.

Foods to eat:

Grape (p.10); Orange (p.16); Prune (p.20); Fig (p.30); Spinach (p.45); Sweet potato (p.50); Almond (p.60); Peanut (p.64); Pumpkin seed (p.67); Whole wheat (p.72); Quinoa (p.75); Lentil (p.77); Kidney bean (p.81); Haddock (p.87); Oyster (p.88); Chicken (p.91); Parsley (p.99); Ginger (p.100); Coconut oil (p.117)

DIGESTIVE COMPLAINTS

Digestive problems don't have to be an inevitable aspect of getting older. The key to keeping the digestive system in good shape is to eat plenty of fibre-rich foods and drink lots of water.

If you suffer from indigestion – discomfort, or a burning feeling in the oesophagus – try to reduce your intake of acid-forming foods, such as cheese and red meat, and eat more foods containing digestive enzymes and fibre.

Foods to eat:

Grape (p.10); Papaya (p.15); Banana (p.19); Blackcurrant (p.22); Grapefruit (p.27); Watercress (p.48); Artichoke (p.49); Brussels sprout (p.54); Carrot (p.57); Almond (p.60); Whole wheat (p.72); Brown rice (p.73); Millet (p.74); Buckwheat (p.76); Chickpea (p.80); Bio-yoghurt (p.95); Garlic (p.98); Ginger (p.100); Fennel (p.102); Dandelion (p.103); Cayenne pepper (p.104); Chamomile (p.105); Cider vinegar (p.115)

VARICOSE VEINS

Varicose veins are twisted, enlarged veins near the surface of the skin, which occur most commonly in the legs and ankles. Normally, the one-way valves in veins keep the blood flowing efficiently against gravity up towards the heart. However, when the valves fail to function properly, blood pools, pressure builds up and the veins become weakened. Vitamin C-rich foods, as well as those containing copper and phenolic compounds are thought to help to prevent varicose veins.

Foods to eat:

Lemon (p.18); Walnut (p.62); Green tea (p.96); Fennel (p.102); Dandelion (p.103)

JOINT PROBLEMS

Keep your joints supple by eating antioxidant-rich fruits and vegetables, along with nuts, seeds and oily fish. Some spices, such as cayenne pepper, may be used topically to help to relieve aching joints.

Foods to eat:

Apple (p.25); Pineapple (p.26); Cherry (p.32); Avocado (p.34); Sesame seed and oil (p.65); Sunflower seed and oil (p.66); Flaxseed (p.68); Lentil (p.77); Salmon (p.84); Herring (p.86); Oyster (p.88); Parsley (p.99); Ginger (p.100); Turmeric (p.101); Fennel (p.102); Cayenne pepper (p.104); Chamomile (p.105); Paprika (p.107); Ginkgo biloba (p.108); Wheatgerm (p.113); Cider vinegar (p.115); Olive oil (p.118)

MEMORY LOSS

As we get older our bodies start to make less of the chemicals our brain cells need to work, thus making it harder to recall stored information. Studies have shown that vitamin E, magnesium and other nutrients may help to counteract this and so prevent memory loss. Researchers are also studying the possibility that foods rich in antioxidants, – particularly vitamins C and E and the mineral silica – might help to keep our brains fit and active in later life.

Foods to eat:

Mango (p.12); Fig (p.30); Beetroot (p.36); Pepper (p.39); Kale (p.43); Spinach (p.45); Cabbage (p.46); Watercress (p.48); Walnut (p.62); Sunflower seed (p.66); Pumpkin seed (p.67); Whole wheat (p.72); Millet (p.74); Salmon (p.84); Prawn (p.85); Herring (p.86); Oyster (p.88); Egg (p.92); Parsley (p.99); Turmeric (p.101); Cayenne pepper (p.104); Ginseng (p.106); Ginkgo biloba (p.108); Wheatgerm (p.113); Olive oil (p.118)

EYE DISEASE

If you want to keep your eyes shiny and bright, remember the old adage about eating your carrots – or, in fact, any brightly coloured fruit and vegetables. Studies suggest that the antioxidants they contain – including vitamins A, C and E and lutein – benefit the eyes by helping the lenses to adjust to changes in light; maintaining the macula (the part of the eye that enables clear vision); and keeping the eyes moist.

Foods to eat:
Apricot (p.13); Blueberry (p.14); Pomegranate (p.31); Cherry (p.32); Beetroot (p.36); Pepper (p.39); Kale (p.43); Pumpkin (p.58); Swiss chard (p.55); Carrot (p.57); Sesame seed (p.65); Barley (p.70); Lamb (p.89); Egg (p.92); Bio-yoghurt (p.95)

OSTEOPOROSIS

Bone loss occurs as we age, and unless we take the right precautions, we can find ourselves suffering from osteoporosis. A diet rich in calcium is critical for maintaining bone strength throughout life, and vitamin D is also important, as it helps the body to absorb calcium.

Foods to eat:
Cucumber (p.37); Broccoli (p.44); Spinach (p.45); Pumpkin seed(p.67); Flaxseed (p.68); Herring (p.86); Haddock (p.87); Oyster (p.88); Milk (p.94); Bio-yoghurt (p.95); Parsley (p.99); Ginger (p.100); Cayenne pepper (p.104); Olive oil (p.118)

HEART DISEASE

Along with taking regular cardiovascular exercise, you can go a long way to keeping your heart healthy by avoiding foods containing saturated fats, which raise your cholesterol levels and clog your arteries. Instead, make sure you use healthy monosaturated oils and eat foods containing flavonoids and plenty of fibre.

Foods to eat:
Grape (p.10); Papaya (p.15); Cranberry (p.17); Cantaloupe melon (p.24); Grapefruit (p.27); Pomegranate (p.31); Avocado (p.34); Pepper (p.39); Onion (p.41); Broccoli (p.44); Cabbage (p.46); Mushroom (p.52); Asparagus (p.53); Swiss chard (p.55); Almond (p.60); Cashew nut (p.63); Peanut (p.64); Flaxseed (p.68); Oats (p.69); Barley (p.70); Soya bean (p.78); Sardine (p.82); Oyster (p.88); Green tea (p.96); Garlic (p.98); Fennel (p.102); Coconut oil (p.117)

glossary

Allicin volatile oil found in garlic that may help to suppress tumours

Alpha-hydroxy-acid (AHA) various fruit acids that are capable of trapping moisture in the skin and initiating the formation of collagen, thus helping to prevent the appearance of wrinkles

Anthocyanins dark purple-coloured pigments that are antioxidant and aid blood flow

Antioxidant compound that inhibits the effects of harmful free radicals

Arginine organic compound found in animal proteins and peanuts

Astringent acts to draw together, constrict and bind and is found in skin preparations

Betacyanin crimson pigment found in beetroot

Bifida bacteria beneficial bacteria that inhabit the intestinal tract and help to fight off infection

Caffeic acid organic acid found in fruits and vegetables

Capsaicin plant chemical found in chilli

Collagen protein central to the maintenance of healthy skin and connective tissue

Conjugated linoleic acid (CLA) naturally occurring fatty acid

Curcumin a potent anti-inflammatory pigment found in turmeric

Cynarin detoxifying, liver-supporting substance

Dimethylaminoethanol (DMAE) chemical compound related to choline, a precursor to the neurotransmitter acetylcholine, and found naturally in fish

Docosahexaenoic acid (DHA) omega-3 fatty acid found in fish oil

Ellagic acid anti-carcinogenic substance found in berries

Ferulic acid antioxidant that protects cells from harmful ultraviolet rays

Flavonoid umbrella term for anti-inflammatory bio-active compounds

Free radicals molecules that damage the body's tissues, produced as a by-product of metabolism or environmental factors

Gamma-linolenic acid (GLA) fatty acid needed for healthy hormone balance, to help lower inflammation and to reduce blood clotting

Glutathione peroxidase enzyme in the body that is a powerful scavenger of free radicals

Hesperidin white or colourless crystalline compound found in citrus fruits

Homocysteine amino acid used normally by the body in cellular metabolism and the manufacture of proteins, but considered a risk factor for several diseases if levels are elevated in the blood

Lactobacillus bacteria, named as such because most of its members convert lactose and other simple sugars to lactic acid

Limonene anti-carcinogenic chemical found in lemons and oranges

Linoleic acid unsaturated fatty acid considered essential to the human diet

Lipoic acid organic acid produced by cells of certain micro-organisms, and essential to processes during metabolism

Lutein antioxidant carotenoid important for eye health

Lycopene antioxidant carotenoid found in red foods

Malic acid tart-tasting organic acid found in apples

Myricetin antioxidant with anti-inflammatory action

Oleic acid oily liquid, and building block for omega-9 fatty acids

Omega-3 and -6 fatty acids polyunsaturated fats found in oily fish, nuts and seeds

Papain enzyme found in papaya that aids protein digestion

Phenethyl isothiocyanate compound found in vegetables that may be anti-carcinogenic

Phytic acid principal storage form of phosphorus in many plant tissues, especially seeds

Phytochemical plant compound with health-giving properties

Phytoestrogen plant compounds with effects similar to but weaker than those of oestrogen

Polyphenol compounds used for chemical synthesis

Quercetin flavonoid with antioxidant properties

Rutin flavonoid for toning and healing peripheral blood vessels

Salicylate salt or ester of salicylic acid; the active substance found in aspirin, and to treat skin conditions

S-allylcysteine compound found in garlic, said to be anti-carcinogenic

Saponins detoxifying, anti-inflammatory compounds found in herbs, pulses and vegetables in the plant's outer layer where they form a protective coating

Sulforaphane anti-carcinogenic compound

Terpenes help to produce enzymes that deactivate carcinogens

Tocotrienol antioxidant that comprises Vitamin E

Zeaxanthin antioxidant carotenoid important for maintaining eye health

index